NEW SYNDROMES

BIRTH DEFECTS: ORIGINAL ARTICLE SERIES

Daniel Bergsma, Series Editor
Volumes in the series published by Alan R. Liss, Inc.

The National Foundation – March of Dimes
Birth Defects: Original Article Series, Volume XIII, Number 3B, 1977

NEW SYNDROMES

Part B of
Annual Review of Birth Defects, 1976

Sponsored by The National Foundation–March of Dimes at
The University of British Columbia
Vancouver, British Columbia, Canada

Editors: **Daniel Bergsma, MD,** Vice President for Professional
Education, The National Foundation

R. Brian Lowry, MB, FRCP(C), Department of Medical
Genetics, University of British Columbia, Vancouver,
British Columbia

Associate Editors: **John M. Opitz, MD,** Professor of Medical Genetics and
Pediatrics, University of Wisconsin, Madison

Natalie W. Paul, The National Foundation

ALAN R. LISS, INC., NEW YORK

To enhance medical communication in the birth defects field, The National Foundation publishes the *Birth Defects Atlas and Compendium,* an *Original Article Series, Syndrome Identification,* a *Reprint Series,* and provides a series of films and related brochures.

Further information can be obtained from:

Professional Education Department
The National Foundation—March of Dimes
1275 Mamaroneck Avenue
White Plains, New York 10605

Published by:

Alan R. Liss, Inc.
150 Fifth Avenue
New York, New York 10011

Library of Congress Cataloging in Publication Data
Main entry under title:

New syndromes

    (Birth defects: original article series; v. 13, no. 3B)
    (Part B of Annual review of birth defects, 1976)
    Includes bibliographical references and index.
    1. Abnormalities, Human—Congresses. 2. Syndromes—Congresses. I. Bergsma, Daniel. II. Lowry, Robert Brian. III. National Foundation. IV. Series. V. Series: Annual review of birth defects, 1976, pt. B [RG626.B63] vol. 13, no. 3B 616'.043'08s [616'043] ISBN 0-8451-1011-X 77-23451

Printed in the United States of America

THE NATIONAL FOUNDATION is dedicated to the long-range goal of preventing birth defects. Our interim goal is to search for ways to ameliorate those birth defects which cannot be prevented.

As a part of our efforts to achieve these goals, we sponsor, or participate in, a variety of scientific meetings and symposia where all questions relating to birth defects are freely discussed. Through our professional educational program we speed the dissemination of information by publishing the proceedings of these meetings and symposia. Now and then, in the course of these discussions, individual participants may express personal viewpoints which go beyond the purely scientific in nature and into controversial matters; abortion for example. It should be noted, therefore, that personal viewpoints about such matters will not be censored but obviously this does not constitute an endorsement of them by The National Foundation.

Contents

CASE REPORTS

Contributors

Pertti Aula [187]
Children's Hospital
University of Helsinki
SF–00290 Helsinki 29
Finland

José María Cantú [139]
Division de Genetica y Hematologia
Unidad de Investigacion
Biomedica de Occidente
Instituto Mexicano del Seguro Social
Apartado Postal 13838
Guadalajara, Jalisco
Mexico

Jaroslav Červenka [1]
Associate Professor
Divisions of Oral Pathology and
Human and Oral Genetics
School of Dentistry
University of Minnesota
Minneapolis, MN 55455

John Chandler [117]
Associate Professor of Ophthalmology
Department of Ophthalmology
University of Washington School
of Medicine
Seattle, WA 98195

M. Michael Cohen, Jr. [1]
Department of Pediatrics
University of Washington School
of Dentistry and Medicine
Seattle, WA 98195

Richard J. Cooke [45]
Department of Pediatrics
University of Virginia
School of Medicine
Charlottesville, VA 22904

John P. Dorst [149]
Division of Medical Genetics
Department of Medicine
The Johns Hopkins University
School of Medicine
Baltimore, MD 21205

Mary Virginia Durkin-Stamm [31]
Department of Medical Genetics
Wisconsin Clinical Genetics Center
University of Wisconsin
Madison, WI 53706

John R. Eastman [39]
Departments of Oral-Facial and
Medical Genetics
Indiana University School of
Dentistry
Indianapolis, IN 46202

B. Rafael Elejalde [53, 103]
Department of Medical Genetics
University of Wisconsin Medical School
Madison, WI 53706

Uta Francke [103, 167]
Department of Pediatrics
University of California
La Jolla, CA 92037

Andrew N. Gale [127]
Division of Medical Genetics
The Johns Hopkins Hospital
Baltimore, MD 21205
Present Address:
8 Rock Mount Close
Liverpool L25 6JN
England

The number in brackets following each contributor's name is the opening page number of that author's paper.

Diana García-Cruz [139]
Division de Genetica y Hematologia
Unidad de Investigacion
  Biomedica de Occidente
Instituto del Seguro Social
Apartado Postal 13838
Guadalajara, Jalisco
Mexico

Nicholas F. Geimer [31]
Internist Hematologist
Department of Medicine
University of Wisconsin Center for
  Health Sciences and Medical School
Madison, WI 53706

Enid F. Gilbert [53]
Departments of Pediatrics and
  Pathology
University of Wisconsin Center for
  Health Sciences and Medical School
Madison, WI 53706

Richard C. Gilmartin [95]
Section of Pediatric Neurology
LeBonheur Children's Hospital
Memphis, TN 38103

Cesar Giraldo [53]
Department of Pathology
Antioquia University
Apartado aero 1226
Medellin, Colombia

Claudette Hajaj Gonzalez [31]
Clinical Genetics Center
Department of Medical Genetics
University of Wisconsin Center for
  Health Sciences and Medical School
Madison, WI 53706

W. Manford Gooch, III [95]
Section of Pediatric Neurology
LeBonheur Children's Hospital
Memphis, TN 38103

Robert J. Gorlin [1]
Professor and Chairman
Division of Oral Pathology
School of Dentistry
University of Minnesota
Minneapolis, MN 55455

Judith G. Hall [117]
Associate Professor
Departments of Pediatrics
  and Medicine
University of Washington School
  of Medicine
Seattle, WA 98105

Mary Jo Harrod [111]
Department of Internal Medicine
University of Texas Health
  Science Center
Dallas, TX 75235

Alejandro Hernández [139]
Instituto Mexicano del Seguro
  Social
Apartado Postal 13838
Guadalajara, Jalisco
Mexico

Jürgen Herrmann [103]
Associate Professor of Pediatrics
  and Medical Genetics
University of Wisconsin Center for
  Health Sciences and Medical School
Madison, WI 53706

David W. Hollister [85]
Division of Medical Genetics
Harbor General Hospital
Torrance, CA 90509

Jorge Howard, Sr. [111]
Department of Pediatrics
University of Texas Health
  Science Center
Dallas, TX 75235

Stanley L. Inhorn [103]
Cytogenetics Laboratory of the
Wisconsin State Laboratory of
Hygiene
Madison, WI 53706

Charles Jackson [117]
Department of Pediatrics
University of Washington School
of Medicine
Seattle, WA 98195

Raul Jimenez [53]
Department of Oral Pathology
Antioquia University
Apartado aereo 1226
Medellin, Colombia

Gilbert Jones [195]
Departments of Pediatrics and
Otolaryngology
University of Tennessee Center
for the Health Sciences
Memphis, TN 38163

Doman K. Keele [111]
Department of Pediatrics
University of Texas Health
Science Center
Dallas, TX 75235

Thaddeus E. Kelly [45, 149]
Department of Pediatrics
University of Virginia
School of Medicine
Charlottesville, VA 22904

Richard W. Kesler [45]
Department of Pediatrics
University of Virginia
School of Medicine
Charlottesville, VA 22904

Yves Lacassie [127]
Division of Medical Genetics
The Moore Clinic
The Johns Hopkins Hospital
Baltimore, MD 21205

Jaakko Leisti [187]
Children's Hospital
University of Helsinki
SF-00290 Helsinki 29
Finland

L. Stefan Levin [127]
Division of Medical Genetics
The Moore Clinic
The Johns Hopkins Hospital
Baltimore, MD 21205

Jack R. Lichtenstein [149]
Department of Dermatology
Washington University School
of Medicine
St. Louis, MO 63110

R. Brian Lowry [203]
Associate Professor
Department of Medical Genetics
The University of British Columbia
Vancouver, BC V5Z 1L7
Canada

John Mann [167]
Department of Pediatrics and
Genetics
The Permanente Medical Group
Santa Clara, CA 95051

Carlos Manzano [139]
Servicio de Radiologia
Hospital de Pediatria
Centro Medico Nacional
Instituto Mexicano del
Seguro Social
Mexico 7 DF, Mexico

Philip D. Mattson [167]
Department of Pediatrics
Southern California Permanente
San Diego, CA 92120

Verna McHaney [195]
Departments of Pediatrics and
Otolaryngology
University of Tennessee Center for
the Health Sciences
Memphis, TN 38163

Victor A. McKusick [127]
Chairman and Physician-in-Chief
Department of Medicine
The Johns Hopkins Hospital
Baltimore, MD 21205

Lorraine F. Meisner [103]
Cytogenetics Laboratory of the
Wisconsin State Laboratory
of Hygiene
Madison, WI 53706

Michael Melnick [39]
Department of Oral-Facial
Genetics
Indiana University Medical Center
Indianapolis, IN 46202

Hans Ochs [117]
Department of Pediatrics
University of Washington School
of Medicine
Seattle, WA 98195

Gary A. Okamoto [117]
Pediatric Fellow
University of Washington School
of Medicine
Seattle, WA 98195

John M. Opitz [31, 103]
Professor of Medical Genetics
and Pediatrics
Department of Medical Genetics
University of Wisconsin School
of Medicine
Madison, WI 53706

Praddy Pagán [139]
Secretaria de Salubridad y
Asistencia
Departmento de Genetica
Hospital Psiquiatrico Infantil
Tlalpan DF
Mexico

Philip D. Pallister [103]
Genetics and Birth Defects Unit
Montana Children's Home and
Hospital
Shodair Crippled Children's Hospital
Helena, MT 59601

David L. Rimoin [85]
Departments of Pediatrics, Medicine
and Radiology
UCLA–Harbor General Hospital
Torrance, CA 90509

Keith Rodaway [117]
Pediatrician
1814 S. 324th Place
Federal Way, WA 98003

John G. Rogers [127]
Division of Medical Genetics
The Moore Clinic
The Johns Hopkins Hospital
Baltimore, MD 21205

Francisco Rubira [31]
Department of Medical Genetics
University of Wisconsin Center
for Health Sciences and
Medical School
Madison, WI 53706
Present Address Unknown

Robert F. Schilling [31]
Professor of Medicine and Hematology
University of Wisconsin Hospitals
Madison, WI 53706

Nasrollah Shahidi [31]
Associate Professor
Department of Pediatrics
University of Wisconsin Medical
School
Madison, WI 53706

Robert S. Sparkes [167]
Division of Medical Genetics
University of California
School of Medicine
Los Angeles, CA 90024

Jürgen Spranger [11, 103]
Chairman, Department of
Pediatrics
University Kinderklinik
65 Mainz, Germany

Emanuel Stadlan [95]
Department of Pathology
University of Tennessee Center
for the Health Sciences
Memphis, TN 38163

Ray E. Stewart [85]
Division of Medical Genetics
UCLA–Harbor General Hospital
Torrance, CA 90509

William Tiddy [103]
Genetics and Birth Defects Unit
Montana Children's Home and
Hospital
Shodair Crippled Children's
Hospital
Helena, MT 59601

David D. Weaver [69]
Department of Medical Genetics
Indiana University School
of Medicine
Indianapolis, IN 46202

Felice Weber [167]
936 Fletcher Lane #12
Hayward, CA 94545

Christopher P. S. Williams [69]
Clinical Director
Child Development and
Rehabilitation Center
Crippled Children's Division
University of Oregon Health
Sciences Center
Portland, OR 97201

Robert S. Wilroy, Jr. [95, 195]
Department of Pediatrics
University of Tennessee Center for
the Health Sciences
Memphis, TN 38163

"Newer" Facial Clefting Syndromes

Robert J. Gorlin, DDS, Jaroslav Červenka, MD, CSc, and M. Michael Cohen, Jr, DMD

In 1970 when asked to present a paper on "Facial Clefting and Its Syndromes," we reported 72 conditions, most being real, while a few were chance associations [1]. During the next five years, while preparing the second edition of "Syndromes of the Head and Neck," we tabulated 117 syndromes of orofacial clefting [2]. This was expanded to 133 conditions by Cohen [3] in 1976; during the last six months of 1976, we have independently gathered another dozen or more, while an additional dozen have been presented in the abstracts of this session. Thus, we estimate about 160 conditions — a few others have been added due to the "chromosomal banding revolution."

One may question whether we are not being too permissive in our criteria for an orofacial clefting syndrome. Does the Down syndrome fall into that category because there is a threefold increase in facial clefting in 21 trisomy (there are two studies which bear this out); do the Waardenburg syndrome, nevoid basal cell carcinoma syndrome, or oculodentoosseous syndrome qualify? Indeed, one finds an association with clefting in these conditions that is greater than expected on the basis of chance. There is obviously no single answer — it depends on the attitude of the one who is doing the tabulation since, in our experience, decision for exclusion or inclusion is frequently arbitrary.

Our intention here is not to be all-inclusive — indeed that would be poor judgment. The reader may elect to peruse either of the above-mentioned works for more comprehensive coverage.

Severe Craniofacial Anomalies and Congenital Amputation or Constrictions of Limbs or Digits

Jones et al [4] and Kubáček and Pěnkava [5] reported several patients with a variety of severe craniofacial anomalies in association with intrauterine amputation, or constriction of limbs, and/or pseudosyndactyly of digits. Survival beyond

Birth Defects: Original Article Series, Volume XIII, Number 3B, pages 1–9

the neonatal period occurred in most cases. Frequency is 1 per 10,000 births and all have been sporadic.

The craniofacial anomalies included severe microcephaly with deficiencies of the anterior calvaria, asymmetric (usually anteriorly located) encephaloceles which are occasionally multiple, microphthalmia with distortion of palpebral fissures, nasal deformities, bizarre facial clefts, and various bands about the face. Less frequent findings were unilateral proboscis, gastroschisis, and talipes equinovarus.

Cleft Palate and Lateral Lingual Pterygia

Unrelated probands have manifested autosomal dominant inheritance of a combination of bilateral mucosal folds extending from the lateral border of the tongue to the free edge of the palatal cleft [6–8]. We believe this to represent a genetic entity distinct from other associations of intraoral synechiae (as in the Hanhart/Möbius syndrome).

Cleft Lip-Palate, Microcephaly, and Hypoplasia of Radius and Thumb

Juberg and Hayward [9] noted cleft lip-palate, microcephaly, hypoplastic and distally positioned thumbs, and shortened radii in three of six sibs. The parents were normal and nonconsanguineous. Similar findings were described by Murphy and Lubin [10].

Cleft Palate and Accessory Metacarpal of Index Finger

Manzke [11] reported a female child with cleft palate, micrognathia, glossoptosis, pectus carinatum, and an accessory metacarpal at the base of the index finger bilaterally, producing clinodactyly. Similar cases were reported by Farnsworth and Pacik [12] and Holthusen [13]. All reported cases have been sporadic.

Cleft Lip-Palate, Hypohidrosis, Thin Wiry Hair, and Dystrophic Nails

Rapp and Hodgkins [14] and Wannarachue et al [15] noted the combination of hypohidrosis, sparse wiry scalp hair, nail dystrophy, short stature, and clefting of the lip and/or palate in a mother and in her son and daughter. Summitt and Hiatt [16] described a white male child with bilateral cleft lip-palate, hypospadias, chordee, sparse and wiry scalp hair, hypohidrosis, nail dysplasia, deficiency of Meibomian glands, few lashes, corneal opacities, photophobia, ectropion of lower lids, slow growth, and slitlike ear canals. An affected mother and her similarly affected children have been observed by Spaulding [17]. A female infant with blond wiry hair, nail dysplasia, frontal bossing, hypohidrosis, and cleft palate was seen by Schorr [18]. This disorder was probably inherited as an autosomal dominant trait.

Moynahan [19] described what he called the "XTE syndrome" in sibs who were the product of a consanguineous union. The syndrome consisted of cleft palate, hypohidrosis and dry skin, nail deformities, dry coarse hair, evanescent cutaneous bullae, absence of lashes on lower lids, small lacrimal puncta, and defective enamel. The relationship of this disorder to those cases described above is unknown.

Fára [20] and Massengill et al [21] each described a female with sparse hair, severe hypodontia, and cleft lip-palate. Watson and Hardwick [22] reported a girl with bilateral cleft lip-palate, hypoplastic pinnas, anodontia, and dystrophic nails. A sib who died soon after birth had cleft lip-palate and a congenital heart defect. The parents were consanguineous; perhaps there is genetic heterogeneity. Some of these cases may be incomplete forms of the EEC syndrome.

Cleft Palate and Lethal Micromelic Dwarfism With Marked Shortness of the Radius and Fibula

De la Chapelle et al [23] reported a unique, apparently recessively inherited form of lethal micromelic dwarfism in a brother and sister whose parents were consanguineous.

Extension of the elbows and knees was limited. The joints were somewhat enlarged and there was talipes equinovarus. The fingers and toes, although normal in number, were very short. The trunk length was reduced and the belly was large. The root of the nose was rather flat, with associated ocular hypertelorism. The ears were low set. Both children had cleft palate.

Roentgenographically, the radius and the fibula were particularly affected, being wide, short, and somewhat triangular. A certain degree of campomelia was present in the femurs and tibias. The proximal portion of the humerus was widened. The bones of the hand were inadequately ossified. The proximal phalanges were not visible, and the middle phalanges were doubled in the boy. The scapulas were abnormally formed. The iliac wings were small. The vertebral bodies were small and unequal, and numerous hemivertebras were present.

Hepatosplenomegaly was present in both children, but only the boy had multiple heterotopic hyperplastic adenomas of the parathyroid and adrenal glands, and hyperplasia of endocrine pancreatic tissue. In addition, both children had patent foramen ovale and ductus arteriosus.

Cleft Palate and Bilateral Femoral and Fibular Dysgenesis

Bailey and Beighton [24], Daentl et al [25], and others [26–29] described patients with femoral and fibular dysgenesis and short stature; several of them had cleft palate. There was mongoloid obliquity of palpebral fissures, short nose with alar hypoplasia, long philtrum, thin upper lip, and micrognathia. In addition, they had dislocated and hypoplastic patellas, hypoplastic pelvis, talipes equinovarus, derangement of elbow joints and lower spine abnormalities. The genetic nature of the syndrome, if it exists, is not known. Patients described by Holthusen [29] may have the same disorder. It has been suggested that this is a variant of the "caudal regression syndrome," since mothers may be diabetic (Optiz, personal communication).

Cleft Palate and Short Stature

Gareis and Smith [30] described a kindred in which several affected members had stature below the third percentile because of relative shortness of the limbs. All affected males and about half the affected females had cleft palate or submucous cleft palate and bifid uvula. Micrognathia was also present in about half of those affected. The condition is dominantly inherited, possibly an X-linked trait.

Cleft Palate and Rüdiger Syndrome

Rüdiger et al [31] described a lethal, probably autosomal recessive syndrome in sibs, the infants succumbing within the first year of life. The disorder is characterized by retardation of psychomotor development, flexion contracture of hands with thick palmar creases, simian lines, small fingers and nails, and ureteral stenosis. Arches were noted on all fingers. The facies were coarse, and the soft palate was cleft.

Cleft Palate, Unusual Facies, Mental Retardation, and Limb Abnormalities

Palant et al [32] described sisters with mild microcephaly, short stature, mental retardation, "almond-shaped, deep-set" eyes, bulbous nasal tip, cleft palate, clinodactyly of toes, and firm, nonbony prominence of the anteromedial aspect of the wrists. The syndrome probably has autosomal recessive inheritance.

Cleft Palate, Macular Coloboma, and Skeletal Abnormality

Phillips and Griffiths [33] reported male and female sibs with bilateral macular coloboma, cleft palate, hallux valgus, retardation of psychomotor development, and flexion deformities of distal interphalangeal joints of the little fingers. The brother was mentally retarded, with dislocation of the patella, coxa valga, and genu valgum.

Cleft Palate and Micrognathic Dwarfism

Maroteaux et al [34] and others [35–37] described a micromelic type of dwarfism characterized by a small mandible and marked widening of the metaphyses of long bones. Cleft vertebras were often visible in the lumbar region, and a slight median fissure of the bony plates was observed in anteroposterior views. Later the development of the epiphyses was insufficient particularly in the femoral heads, and growth was slow. The disorder appears to have autosomal recessive inheritance. Cleft palate was present in all those affected.

Haller et al [37] reported that, with time, the long bones show normal length and almost normal form. Thoracic platyspondyly was evident, and the 2nd lumbar vertebra was kyphotic.

Recurrent Brachial Plexus Neuritis and Cleft Palate

Erikson [38] reported a syndrome in a father and his two daughters. The syndrome was characterized by sudden attacks of pain in the shoulder which radiated to the arms and hands. The pain gradually disappeared, but paresthesia and weakness in the upper limbs were noted. There was also limitation of extension at the elbow and winging of the scapulas. Sensory loss over the hand and forearm was evident. An electromyogram revealed partial denervation of several muscles of the arm and hand, the distribution being compatible with a lesion of the brachial plexus. The neuritis initially appeared at age three or four years.

In all three individuals the face was unusual. There was facial asymmetry and mild mongoloid obliquity of the palpebral fissures and the eyes appeared deeply and closely set. All three patients had cleft palate. Other patients exhibiting brachial neuritis, similar facies, and cleft palate were reported by Jacob et al [39]. Similar facies were evident in the cases of Poffenbarger [40] and Gardner and Maloney [41]. The syndrome was inherited in an autosomal dominant manner.

Microcephaly, Large Ears, Short Stature, and Cleft Palate

Say et al [42] reported a dominantly inherited syndrome in which cleft palate was associated with small head size, large ears, and short stature. The patient's mother and sister had tapered fingers with hypoplastic distal phalanges involving the 2nd to 4th digits bilaterally, ulnar deviation of the middle fingers, low-set thumbs and bilateral acromial dimples.

Cleft Palate and Kniest Syndrome

The disorder described by Kniest [43] in 1952 is a rare form of disproportionate dwarfism, often confused with the Morquio syndrome or metatropic dwarfism. Although nearly all cases have been sporadic, Maroteaux and Spranger [44] observed the syndrome in a mother and daughter.

The face is round, with flat midface and depressed nasal bridge, giving the eyes an exophthalmic appearance. The neck is short and the head appears to sit upon the thorax. At birth, the patient is frequently noted to have cleft palate, clubfoot, and prominent knees. Lordosis and/or kyphoscoliosis and tibial bowing usually develop within the first few years of age, respectively. By that time, most joints become progressively enlarged, stiff, and painful. Movement at the metacarpophalangeal joint is normal, but the child cannot make a fist. The 5th fingers are generally not involved. The elbows and wrists become especially enlarged, and flexion and extension of most joints become progressively reduced. Gait is markedly altered. Adult height ranges between 105 and 145 cm.

Severe myopia and lattice degeneration with or without retinal detachment and/or cataract formation have been present in less than half of reported cases, as has cleft palate. Conduction and/or sensorineural deafness may develop before puberty. Recurrent respiratory infections are common.

Roentgenographically, the neurocranium is large compared to the facial skeleton. Platyspondyly, especially of the upper thoracic vertebras, is severe. The interpedicular distances in the lumbar portion of the spine narrow sacrally. The bones of the upper limbs are short. The metaphyses of long bones flare, and the epiphyses are large, irregular, and punctate.

The proximal row of carpal bones is small, especially in relation to the large capital femoral epiphysis and proximal femoral metaphysis. The femoral capital epiphysis forms late, the neck is wide and short with a poorly ossified central area, and there may be coxa vara. The trochanter is prominent.

Histopathologic examination of the bones has shown large chondrocytes which lie in a very loosely woven matrix containing numerous empty spaces ("Swiss cheese cartilage") [45].

Miscellaneous Clefting Syndromes

Bowen and Armstrong [46] reported an autosomal recessive syndrome of cleft lip-palate with growth and mental retardation, areas of hyperpigmented skin, filiform adhesion of eyelids, oligodontia, and syndactyly of toes [2–5].

Pallister et al [47], using the term "W syndrome," reported incomplete cleft of lip and of anterior hard palate in combination with prematurity, marked mental retardation, seizures, high forehead, downward slanting palpebral fissures, broad nasal tip, strabismus, missing maxillary central incisors, cubitus valgus, and various minor skeletal anomalies. Inheritance is probably X-linked with mild expression in female heterozygotes, but may also be autosomal dominant.

Fontaine et al [48] described autosomal dominant inheritance of cleft palate or submucous cleft palate with micrognathia, dysplastic ears, ectrodactyly, and syndactyly (feet), with mental retardation in some cases.

Ho et al [49] noted a child with micrognathia, wormian bones, dislocated hips, absent tibias, bowed fibulas, preaxial polydactyly of feet, ulnar deviation of fingers, simian creases, and congenital heart anomaly.

Fitch and Levy [50] reported another case of cleft palate with microcephaly and adducted thumbs, a syndrome reviewed earlier by Gorlin et al [1].

Hay and Wells [51] described autosomal dominant inheritance of cleft lip-palate, ankyloblepharon, hair loss, absent or dystrophic nails, partial anhidrosis, lacrimal duct atresia, supernumerary nipples, syndactyly, and teeth with conical crowns.

Clefting and Chromosomal Aneuploidy

In addition to the oft-quoted association of clefting with trisomy 13 (60–80%), trisomy 18 (15%), and trisomy 21 (1 per 200), our analysis of the recent literature would suggest a more than chance association of cleft lip and cleft palate with the following chromosomal disorders: 3p+ [2, 52], 4p– [2], 7q+ [2, 53, 54], 8+ [55], 10p+ [56–58], 10q+ [2, 57, 58], 11p+ [2], 11q+ [59, 60], 13q– [2, 61], 14q+ [62], 18p– [2], 18q– [2], 19q+ [63], 21q– [2], 22+ [2, 64–66], XXXXY [2], and triploidy [2, 67]. As we write this, we have little doubt that this list is already obsolete.

REFERENCES

1. Gorlin RJ, Cervenka J, Pruzansky S: Facial clefting and its syndromes. In Bergsma D (ed): Part XI. "Orofacial Structures." Baltimore: Williams & Wilkins for The National Foundation–March of Dimes, BD:OAS VII(7):3–49, 1971.
2. Gorlin RJ, Pindborg JJ, Cohen MM Jr: "Syndromes of the Head and Neck." 2nd Ed. New York: McGraw-Hill, 1976.
3. Cohen MM Jr: Syndromes with cleft lip and palate. J Oral Surg. (In press.)
4. Jones KL, Smith DW, Hall BD, Hall JG, Ebbin AJ, Massoud H, Golbus MS: A pattern of craniofacial and limb defects secondary to aberrant tissue bands. J Pediatr 84:90–95, 1974.
5. Kubaček V, Pěnkava J: Oblique clefts of the face. Acta Chir Plast (Praha) 16:152–163, 1974.
6. Berendes J: Angeborene Synechie zwischen der Mundbodenschleimhaut und den Oberkieferfortsätzen am Rande einer Gaumenspalt. HNO 9:180–182, 1961.
7. Fuhrmann W: Autosomal dominate Vererbung von Gaumenspalte und Synechien zwischen Gaumen und Mendboden oder Zunge. Humangenetik 14:196–203, 1972.
8. Bartsocas CS: Personal communication, 1974.
9. Juberg RC, Hayward JR: A new familial syndrome of oral, cranial, and digital anomalies. J Pediatr 74:755–762, 1969.
10. Murphy S, Lubin B: Triphalangeal thumbs and congenital erythroid hypoplasia. J Pediatr 81:987–989, 1972.
11. Manzke H: Symmetrische Hyperphalangie des zweiten Fingers durch ein akzessorisches Metacarpale. Fortschr Geb Roentgenstr Nuklearmed 105:425–427, 1966.
12. Farnsworth PB, Pacik PT: Glossoptotic hypoxia and micrognathia: The Pierre-Robin syndrome reviewed. Clin Pediatr 10:600–606, 1971.
13. Holthusen W: The Pierre-Robin syndrome: Unusual associated developmental defects. Ann Radiol (Paris) 15:253–262, 1972.
14. Rapp RS, Hodgkins WE: Anhidrotic ectodermal dysplasia: Autosomal dominant inheritance with palate and lip anomalies. J Med Genet 5:269–272, 1968.
15. Wannarachue N, Hall BD, Smith DW: Ectodermal dysplasia and multiple defects (Rapp-Hodgkins type). J Pediatr 81:1217–1218, 1972.
16. Summitt RL, Hiatt RL: Hypohidrotic ectodermal dysplasia with multiple associated anomalies. In "Orofacial Structures," op cit pp 121–124.
17. Spaulding P: Personal communication, 1975.

18. Schorr WF: Personal communication, 1974.
19. Moynahan E: XTE (xeroderma, talipes and enamel defect): A new heredofamilial syndrome. Two cases: Homozygous inheritance of a dominant gene. Proc R Soc Med 63:447–448, 1970.
20. Fára M; Regional ectodermal dysplasia with total bilateral cleft. Acta Chir Plast (Praha), 13:100–105, 1971.
21. Massengill R, Maxwell S, Quinn G, Pickrell K: An abnormal speech pattern associated with an orofacial anomaly. Acta Otolaryngol (Stockh), 68:537–542, 1969.
22. Watson RM, Hardwick CE: Hypodontia associated with cleft palate. Br Dent J 130:77–80, 1971.
23. De la Chapelle A, Maroteaux P, Haru N, Granroth G: Une rare dysplasie osseuse léthale de transmission recessive autosomique. Arch Fr Pédiatr 29:759–770, 1972.
24. Bailey JA, Beighton P: Bilateral femoral dysgenesis. Clin Pediatr 9:668–674, 1970.
25. Daentl DL, Smith DW, Scott CI, Hall BD, Gooding CA: Femoral hypoplasia – unusual facies syndrome. J Pediatr 86:107–111, 1975.
26. Frantz CH, O'Rahilly R: Congenital skeletal limb deficiencies. J Bone Joint Surg 43A:1218–1224, 1961.
27. Kučera J, Lenz W, Maier W: Missbildungen der Beine und der kaudalen Wirbelsäule bei Kindern diabetischer Mütter. Dtsch Med Wochenschr 90:901–905, 1965.
28. Passarge E: Congenital malformation and maternal diabetes. Lancet 1:324–325, 1965.
29. Holthusen W: The Pierre-Robin syndrome: Unusual associated developmental defects. Ann Radiol (Paris) 15:253–262, 1972.
30. Gareis FJ, Smith DW: Diminished stature-defective palate syndrome: A dominantly inherited disorder. J Pediatr 79:470–472, 1971.
31. Rüdiger RA, Schmidt W, Loose DA, Passarge E: Severe developmental failure with coarse facial features, distal limb hypoplasia, thickened palmar creases, bifid uvula and ureteral stenosis: A previously undescribed familial disorder with lethal outcome. J Pediatr 79:977–981, 1971.
32. Palant DI, Feingold M, Berkman MD: Unusual facies, cleft palate, mental retardation and limb abnormalities in siblings – a new syndrome. J Pediatr 78:686–689, 1971.
33. Phillips CI, Griffiths DL: Macular coloboma and skeletal abnormality. Br J Ophthalmol 53:346–349, 1969.
34. Maroteaux P, Roux C, Fruchter Z: Le nanisme micrognathe. Nouv Presse Méd 78:2371–2374, 1970.
35. Rolland JC, Laugier J, Michel J, Grenier B, Desbuquois G: Un nanisme chondrodystrophique avec division palatine. Arch Fr Pédiatr 27:331, 1970.
36. Weissenbacher G, Zweymüller E: Gleichzeitiges Vorkommen eines Syndroms von Pierre-Robin und einer fetalen Chondrodysplasie. Monatsschr Kinderheilkd 112:315–317, 1964.
37. Haller JO, Berdon WE, Robinow M, Slovis TL, Baker DH, Johnson GF: The Weissenbacher-Zweymüller syndrome of micrognathism and rhizomelic chondrodysplasia at birth with subsequent normal growth. Am J Roentgenol Radium Ther Nucl Med 125:936–943, 1975.
38. Erikson A: Hereditary syndrome consisting in recurrent attacks resembling brachial plexus neuritis, special facial features, and cleft palate. Acta Paediatr Scand 63:885–888, 1964.
39. Jacob JC, Andermann F, Robb JP: Heredofamilial neuritis with brachial predilection. Neurology (Minneap) 11:1025–1033, 1961.
40. Poffenbarger AL: Heredofamilial neuritis with brachial predilection. W Va Med J 64:425–529, 1968.
41. Gardner JH, Maloney W: Hereditary brachial and cranial neuritis. Genetically linked with ocular hypotelorism and syndactyly. Neurology (Minneap) 18:278, 1968.

42. Say B, Barber DH, Hobbs J, Coldwell, JG: A new dominantly inherited syndrome of cleft palate. Humangenetik 26:267–269, 1975.
43. Kniest W: Zur Abgrenzung der Dysostosis enchondralis von der Chondrodystrophie. Z Kinderheilkd 70:633–640, 1952.
44. Maroteaux P, Spranger J; La maladie de Kniest. Arch Fr Pédiatr 30:735–750, 1973.
45. Rimoin D: Histopathology and ultrastructure of cartilage in the chondrodystrophies. In Bergsma D (ed): "Skeletal Dysplasias." Miami: Symposia Specialists for The National Foundation–March of Dimes, BD:OAS X(9):1–18, 1974.
46. Bowen P, Armstrong HB: Ectodermal dysplasia, mental retardation, cleft lip/palate, and other anomalies in three sibs. Clin Genet 9:35–42, 1976.
47. Pallister PD, Herrmann J, Spranger JW, Gorlin RJ, Langer LO, Opitz JM: The W syndrome. In Bergsma D (ed): "Malformation Syndromes." Miami: Symposia Specialists for The National Foundation–March of Dimes, BD:OAS X(7):51–60, 1974.
48. Fontaine G, Farriaux JP, Delattre P, Gidlecki Z, Poúpard B, Piquet J, Durieux G: Une observation familiale du syndrome ectrodactylie et dysostose mandibulo-faciale. J Génét Hum 22:289–307, 1974.
49. Ho CK, Kaufman RL, McAlister WA: Congenital malformations: Cleft palate, congenital heart disease, absent tibiae, and polydactyly. Am J Dis Child 129:714–716, 1975.
50. Fitch N, Levy EP: Adducted thumbs syndrome(s). Clin Genet 8:190–198, 1975.
51. Hay RJ, Wells RS: The syndrome of ankyloblepharon, ectodermal defects, and cleft lip and palate: An autosomal dominant condition. Br J Dermatol 94:277–289, 1976.
52. Allerdice PW, Browne N, Murphy DP: Chromosome 3 duplication q21 → qter in children of carriers of a pericentric inversion inv (3) (p23q21). Am J Hum Genet 27:699–718, 1975.
53. Al Saadi A, Maghadan HA: Partial trisomy of the long arm of chromosome 7. Clin Genet 9:250–254, 1976.
54. Turleau C, Rossier A, de Montis G, Roubin M, Chavin-Colin F, de Grouchy J: Trisomie partielle 7q. Ann Génét-(Paris) 19:37–42, 1976.
55. Riccardi VM: Trisomy 8: An international study of 70 patients. This volume.
56. Nakagome Y, Kobayashi H: Trisomy of the short arm of chromosome 10. J Med Genet 12:412–414, 1975.
57. Yunis E, Silva R, Giraldo A: Trisomy 10p. Ann Génét (Paris) 19:57–60, 1976.
58. Kroyer S, Niebuhr E: Partial trisomy 10q occurring in a family with a reciprocal translocation t(10;18) (q25;q23). Ann Génét (Paris) 18:50–55, 1975.
59. Giraud F, Matter JF, Matter MG, Bernard R: Trisomie partielle 11q et translocation familiale 11-22. Humangenetik 28:343–347, 1975.
60. Auris A, Laurent C: Trisomie 11q. Individualization d'un nouveau syndrome. Ann Génét (Paris) 18:189–191, 1975.
61. Kučerova M, Polivková Z, Pokorná M: Deletion of the long arms of chromosome 13. Humangenetik 27:255–257, 1975.
62. Raoul O, Rethoré MO, Dutrillaux B, Michon L, Lejeune J: Trisomie 14q partielle. I. Trisomie 14q partielle par translocation maternelle t(10;14) (p15;q22). Ann Génét (Paris) 18:35–39, 1975.
63. Lange M, Alfi OS: Trisomy 19q. Ann Génét (Paris) 19:17–21, 1976.
64. Penchaszadeh VB, Coco R: Trisomy 22. Two new cases and delineation of the phenotype. J Med Genet 12:193–199, 1975.
65. Zellweger H, Ionasescu V, Simpson J: Trisomy 22. J Génét Hum 23:65–75, 1975.
66. Vianello MG, Bonioli E: Trisomy 22. J Génét Hum 23:239–250, 1975.
67. Wertelecki W, Graham JM Jr, Sergovich FR: The clinical syndrome of triploidy. Obstet Gynecol 47:69–76, 1976.

"New" Dwarfing Syndromes

Jürgen Spranger, MD

The number of apparently "new" dwarfing conditions reported in the last years is perplexing. A few disorders in some nosologically particularly interesting areas of growth failure will be presented.

General Considerations

The most common cause of small stature is normal variation, leading either to permanent or, in the case of delayed development, to temporary smallness (Fig. 1). By statistical definition, 0.5% of the normal population is very small ($< 3\delta$).

Pathologic forms of dwarfism can be divided into primary and secondary types. In secondary dwarfism the skeleton reacts unfavorably to an extraskeletal disturbance. Its growth potential is normal. Figure 2 demonstrates the striking ability of the skeleton to resume its growth once the extraskeletal disturbance has been removed. In primary dwarfism the growth potential of the skeleton is impaired. Primary dwarfism can be subdivided into three forms: skeletal hypoplasias, dysostoses, and dysplasias.

Skeletal hypoplasias are growth disorders of all tissue components of bone. The skeleton is small, its form and structure is normal, and the dwarfism is more or less proportionate. Dysostoses are developmental defects of single bones, alone or in combination. Dysplasias are systemic disorders of single components of the skeletal tissue. In contrast to the hypoplasias, some components are unaffected. Form and/or structure of the skeleton are abnormal and the resulting dwarfism is usually disproportionate. A skeletal hypoplasia is a nonspecific finding in a great number of chromosomal, mono- or polygenic disorders. One interesting

Birth Defects: Original Article Series, Volume XIII, Number 3B, pages 11–29
© 1977 The National Foundation

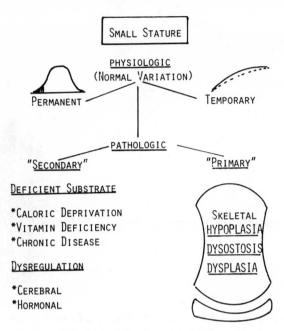

Fig. 1. Classification of dwarfism.

subgroup is that of primordial dwarfism. The term "primordial dwarfism,"* meaning "dwarfism ab ovo" (primordium = origin), was introduced in 1902 by Hansemann [1]. It designates a group of children who are small for date at birth, remain very small and, in most instances, exhibit a number of more or less characteristic dysmorphic signs [2–6]. It is this association of intrauterine growth retardation with a spectrum of phenotypic anomalies that differentiates the various types of primordial dwarfism from nonspecific intrauterine growth retardation. The latter occurs in approximately 0.17% of all children but only rarely results in true dwarfism [7, 8]. Table 1 lists some well-defined types of *primordial dwarfism.* The two following disorders have recently been added to that list.

The MMM Syndrome

The 3 M syndrome was recently described by Miller et al [9]. Its main clinical features are depicted in Figure 3. The 3 M syndrome may be suspected in

---

*In the American literature the term "primordial dwarfism" is sometimes used for sexual ateliosis due to isolated growth hormone deficiency. This use does not correspond to the original definition nor to that of the Paris Classification of Constitutional Diseases of Bone.

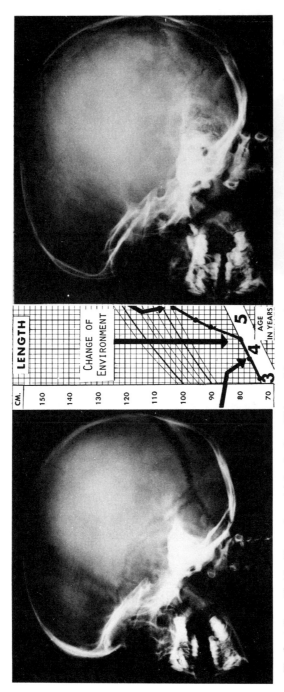

Fig. 2. A 5-yr-old girl with psychosocial deprivation. Wide cranial sutures at the age of 3.5 yr suggested an intracranial tumor. Appropriate studies were negative. The child was placed in a foster home. Without any other measures a rapid growth spurt occurred and the cranial abnormalities disappeared reflecting the normal growth potential of the skeleton in secondary dwarfism.

TABLE 1. Types of Primordial Dwarfism

Syndromes	Prominent Feature	Mental retardation	Genetics
Silver-Russell syndrome	Pseudohydrocephaly (Asymmetry)	φ	?
Bloom syndrome	Facial erythema	φ	AR
Dubowitz syndrome	Eczema, distinct face	±	AR
Bird-headed dwarfs	Microcephaly, Micrognathia	±	AR
Mulibrey nanism	Constrictive pericarditis	φ	AR
Cockayne syndrome	Retinal atrophy	+	AR
Fetal alcohol syndrome	Short palpebral fissures	+	NH
MMM syndrome	Silver-Russell without pseudohydrocephalus	φ	AR

AR = autosomal recessive
NH = nonhereditary

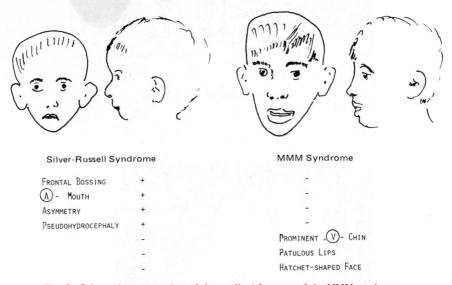

Silver-Russell Syndrome

FRONTAL BOSSING   +
Ⓐ - MOUTH   +
ASYMMETRY   +
PSEUDOHYDROCEPHALY   +
                            -
                            -
                            -

MMM Syndrome

                            -
                            -
                            -
                            -
PROMINENT Ⓥ - CHIN
PATULOUS LIPS
HATCHET-SHAPED FACE

Fig. 3. Schematic presentation of the cardinal features of the MMM syndrome.

a patient resembling a Russell-Silver dwarf but it lacks asymmetry, pseudohydro-cephaly or altered patterns of sexual development. The face is somewhat different in the two conditions; a more prominent chin, patulous lips, and hatchet-shaped profile are present in the 3 M syndrome. In Russell-Silver dwarfism, the face tends to normalize with age [10], whereas, the facial abnormalities in the 3 M syndrome seem to persist [11]. The clinical differentiation of the two syndromes is genetically important. The 3 M syndrome is inherited as an autosomal recessive trait. The Russell-Silver syndrome is almost invariably sporadic and may be an autosomal dominant trait [12].

Brachymelic Seckel Dwarfism

A controversial subgroup of primordial dwarfism is the bird-headed Virchow-Seckel type. Seckel [13] analyzed 2 personal cases and 13 cases from the literature but only his first case corresponded to the usual definition of the Seckel dwarf: A child with intrauterine growth retardation, a small head, small chin, prominent beaked nose, mental retardation, sparse hair, and various congenital anomalies.

Bass et al [14] recently described a patient with these features. In addition, their patient had short limbs with radiographic changes of the proximal limbs. We observed a strikingly similar patient who was the offspring of a consanguineous marriage [15]. There was severe under ossification of the proximal portions of the femora and humeri with resulting shortness of the limbs. Possibly these features were overlooked in previous cases of bird-headed dwarfism. On the other hand, so-called bird-headed dwarfism may be heterogeneous with at least a normal- and a short-limbed type.

The diagnosis of so-called bird-headed dwarfism rests heavily on the head size which is small for height. However, a small head is a nonspecific finding in primordial dwarfism and not every small-headed primordial dwarf is a Seckel dwarf. One example is the fetal alcohol syndrome [16]. Another example is shown in Figure 4 – a 5-yr-old patient with an unclassifiable type of primordial dwarfism characterized by intrauterine and postnatal dwarfism, microcephaly, mental retardation, microdontia, genital hypoplasia, and muscular hypotonia.

In the case of bone dysplasias, there are a few conditions in which the skeletal dysplasia, though prominent, is only part of a wide spectrum of mesenchymal and extramesenchymal disturbances.

Pseudoleprechaunism

Dr. Patterson, at the first Birth Defects Conference in Baltimore, presented a patient as an example of leprechaunism [17]. There were severe bone changes not usually seen in that disorder, and in spite of some clinical similarities to leprechaunism it was suspected that the reported case represented a different entity. Recently, a second patient was observed in Bristol by Dr. David [18]. Although the patients are not dwarfed, they are mentioned here because of their unusual skeletal dysplasia.

The most prominent clinical features are listed in Table 2 and illustrated in Figure 5A. Radiographically, the skeletal maturation is grotesquely delayed with complete lack of epiphyseal ossification at the age of 9 years (Fig. 5B). In addition.

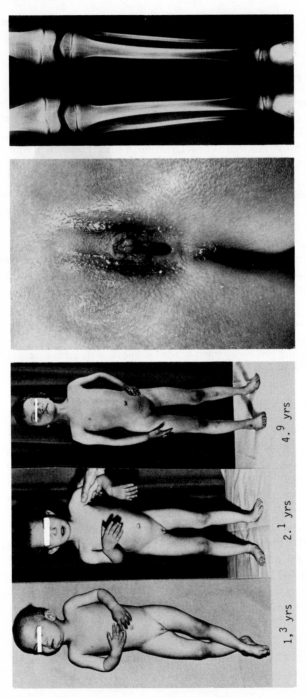

Fig. 4. Clinical aspect of a 5-yr-old girl with an unclassifiable type of microcephalic primordial dwarfism. Her birthweight was 2,250 gm, birth length 46 cm. She failed to thrive and had multiple cerebral seizures. Muscular hypotonia gradually improved. Findings at 5 yr showed a height of 98 cm (below 3rd%), weight of 11 kg (below 3rd%), and head circumference of 45 cm (2nd% for height). Her developmental age was 3 years with considerable speech problems and moderate muscular hypotonia. Further findings included a triangular face, microdontia, and genital hypoplasia. Results of chromosome and extensive biochemical studies, including estrogen and ketosteroid determinations, were normal. The family history was unremarkable. A skeletal survey showed thin shafts of the tubular bones and exostoses in the proximal portions of both fibulas.

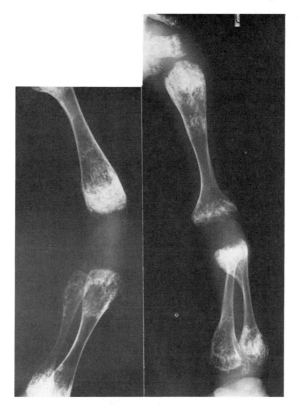

Fig. 5. Dr. David's 9-yr-old patient with pseudoleprechaunism. Complete lack of epiphyseal ossification, severe disturbances of metaphyseal ossification.

TABLE 2. Major Findings in Two Patients With Pseudoleprechaunism

Findings	Patterson's Case [17]	David's Case [18]
Age, sex	7M	9F
Leprechaun face	+	+
Dark skin	+	+
Loose skin	+	+
Excessive hair	+	+
Sexual precocity	+	+
Diabetes mellitus	+	+?
Hyperadrenocorticism	+	?
Mental retardation	+	+
Seizures	+	+
Bone dysplasia	+	+

the metaphyseal ossification is severely disturbed with splayed bone ends and irregular calcific inclusions reaching deep into the diaphyses. The patients appear to suffer from a grave disorder affecting primarily the connective tissue and the (neuro-?)endocrine system.

Multiple Epiphyseal Dysplasia and Diabetes Mellitus

Another disorder with associated skeletal and endocrine abnormalities was described in 1972 by Wolcott and Rallison [19]. They reported three sibs with multiple epiphyseal dysplasia and infancy-onset diabetes mellitus (Table 3). Diabetes mellitus is found very rarely under one year of age. Less than 0.4% of all juvenile diabetics are affected since infancy [19]. Its occurrence in three sibs and its association with a bone disorder is highly unusual and points to a common pathogenesis.

We recently observed a 7-year-old patient with identical bone changes and diabetes mellitus since 10 weeks of age. His sister was diabetic since age 8 weeks and had mild hip changes at 11 months. The clinical and radiographic changes are shown in Figure 6 (A–F). Unfortunately, no thyroid function studies were done, and the possibility of a combined thyroid and pancreatic β-cell deficiency cannot be ruled out. I do not have a unifying concept to explain this familial syndrome of associated skeletal and endocrine defects.

Dwarfism and Humoral Immunodeficiency

In discussing the association of bone dysplasias with other developmental errors, I should like to complement a table with dwarfism-immunodeficiency syndromes presented at last year's conference [20]. Dr. Ammann et al [21] described sibs with dwarfism, a skeletal dysplasia, and deficient antibody-mediated immunity. Dr. Herrmann observed a 2-year-old dwarfed patient with repeated severe respiratory infections, decreased IgG and IgA levels, normal T-cell func-

TABLE 3. Syndrome of Multiple Epiphyseal Dysplasia and Diabetes Mellitus

Findings	Wolcott and Rallison			Personal Observations	
Age, sex	4M	2F	1M	7M	1F
M.E.D.	+	?	+	+	(+)
Infancy-onset diabetes mellitus	+	+	+	+	+
"Dry skin"		+	+	+	
Waddling gait	+			+	
Limit mobility	+			+	φ
Mental retardation				+	+
Seizures	φ	+	φ	φ	φ
Bone fractures	+	φ	φ	φ	φ

tion, and a metaphyseal chondrodysplasia (Fig. 7). An apparently similar patient was shown to me by Dr. C. Carter (London). Thus, the spectrum of dwarfism-immunodeficiency syndromes appears to comprise one disorder with a cell-mediated, one with an antibody-mediated, and one with a combined immuno-deficiency (Table 4). In the latter, a deficient action of the enzyme adenosine deaminase has been repeatedly found. The skeletal changes in the various disorders are markedly similar pointing to similar pathogenetic mechanisms. It may be worthwhile to investigate the activities of other enzymes involved in purine/pyrimidine metabolism in these disorders.

G_{M1} β-Galactosidase Deficiencies

The best known phenotype caused by $G_{M1}\beta$-galactosidase deficiency is that of G_{M1} gangliosidosis type I. Its symptoms appear in the first 6 months of life with a Hurler phenotype, dysostosis multiplex, and hepatosplenomegaly. CNS deterioration is rapid and death usually occurs by age 2 years [22]. In G_{M1} gangliosidosis type II the symptoms appear later, neurologic deterioration is less rapid, viscero-megaly is absent, the bone changes are mild, and death occurs between 3 and 10

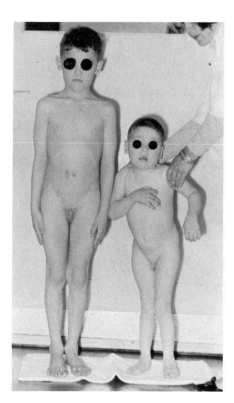

Fig. 6A. A 7-yr-old patient with multiple epiphyseal dysplasia and infancy-onset diabetes mellitus (right); normal control (left). (For clinical description, see Table 3.)

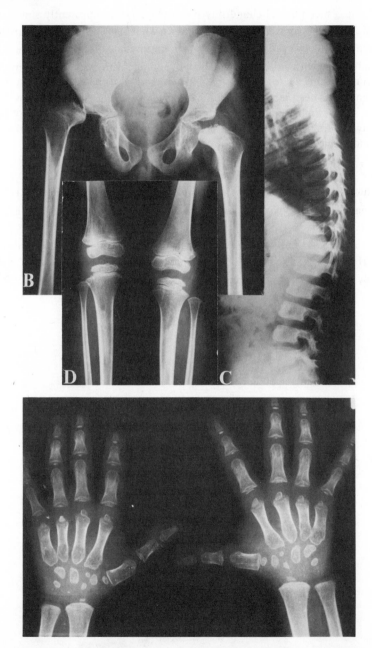

Figs. 6B–E. The epiphyseal ossification is delayed and irregular. There is generalized, mild flattening of the vertebral bodies. The contours of the carpal bones are irregular. Multiple cone-shaped epiphyses are seen in the phalanges.

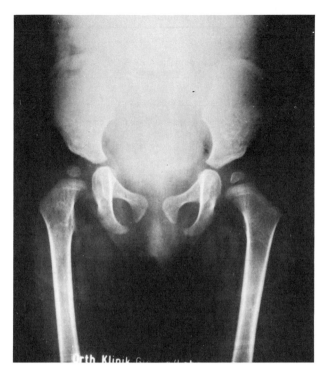

Fig. 6F. The patient's sister at 2 yr. The capital femoral epiphyses are small and the acetabular fossae are shallow.

years of age (Table 5). Whereas in these two types, the skeletal changes are only a relatively minor manifestation of the disease, they are quite prominent or even the leading symptom in a third group of patients.

In type III patients the bone disorder is usually described as a spondylo-epiphyseal dysplasia (Figs. 8 and 9). Usually, it is associated with ocular symptoms and with signs of central nervous system involvement (Table 5). Hurler-like clinical features appear only late, if at all (Figs. 10A and B). The neurologic picture is variable. Ataxia, nystagmus, and other signs of cerebellar dysfunction usually develop between the 4th and 10th year of life [13, 23–28]. Cerebral seizures and spasticity are occasionally seen [13, 26, 28]. After the age of 10 years, myoclonus develops frequently [24–27, 29]. Most patients are mentally defective [23–30].

TABLE 4. Immunodeficiency-Dwarfism Syndromes

Findings	Cartilage-hair hypoplasia	Ammann syndrome	Adenosine deaminase deficiency
Deficient cell-mediated immunity	±	−	++
Deficient antibody-mediated immunity	−	+	++
Brittle hair	+	−	?
Chronic candidiasis	−	−	+
Chronic diarrhea	±	−	+
Recurrent sinopulmonary infections	−	+	+
Severe varicella/vaccinia	+	−	?
Failure to thrive	−	−	++

TABLE 5. Common Types of β-Galactosidase Deficiency

Symptoms	I (Infantile)	II (Juvenile)	III (Adult)
Manifestation (yr)	0.6	1−2	3−8
CNS-deterioration	Rapid	Slower	Slow
Skeletal dysplasia	Marked	Mild	Distinct
Hepatosplenomegaly	Marked	No	No
Corneal opacities	Yes/No	No	Yes
Cherry-red macular spot	Yes/No	No	Yes/No
Vacuolized lymphocytes	Yes	Yes	Yes
β-Galactosidase activity	~1%	~3%	~5−10%
Prognosis	ℵ2 yr	ℵ 10 yr	Survival

Unfortunately, the nosology of G_{M1} β-galactosidase deficiency is more complicated than suggested by the above classification. There are a number of patients who cannot be classified within this scheme. Thus, cases have been described with definite features of G_{M1} gangliosidosis type I such as early onset, rapid neurologic deterioration, and hepatosplenomegaly but without the mesenchymal changes usually seen in that type [31, 32]. Maroteaux [33] described patients with a somewhat different neurologic symptomatology, namely marked extrapyramidal (mostly athetoid) symptoms, normal or almost normal mentation, and no cere-bellar signs. O'Brien et al [34] observed a 15-year-old girl with a distinct spondy-loepiphyseal dysplasia but with normal neurologic function.

The variability of the G_{M1} β-galactoside deficiency phenotype (Fig. 11) is not unexpected in view of the molecular properties of the enzyme [35]. The differences between the three common types are thought to reflect varying residual activities of G_{M1} β-galactosidase toward all the natural substrates [35]. Types I and II are probably caused by allelic mutations and the usual adult type by a nonallelic mutation [36].

Furthermore, variability can be expected from different residual activities for different natural substrates of the enzyme. β-Galactosidase has a great number of

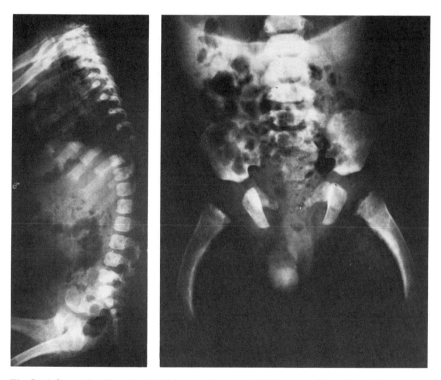

Fig. 7. A 9-month-old patient with humoral immunodeficiency and bone dysplasia (Courtesy Dr. J. Herrmann, Madison, Wis.). The anterior rib ends are flared and concave. The ilia are squared and short in their vertical diameter. The ossification of the proximal femora is delayed and the metaphyseal margins are slightly irregular. There is external bowing of the femoral shafts. The skeletal changes are similar to those described in adenosine deaminase deficiency but there was no abnormality of the T-cell system in this patient.

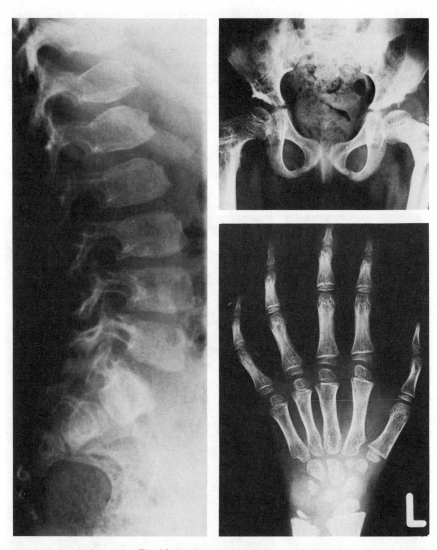

Fig. 8. A 9-yr-old (see also Fig. 10A). The vertebral bodies are flattened, ovoid, and dorsally wedged. The lower portions of the ilia are hypoplastic with an increased flare of the iliac wings. The acetabula are shallow. A bilateral subtrochanteric osteotomy has been preformed. The 2nd–5th metacarpals are proximally pointed; the carpal bones are irregular and the planes of the distal radial and ulnar growth plates are slanted toward one another. The bone trabeculation is prominent and irregular.

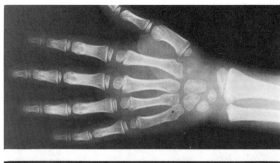

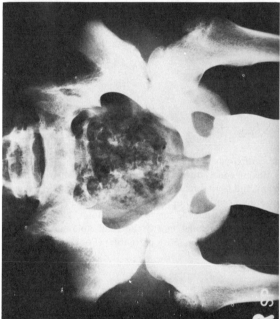

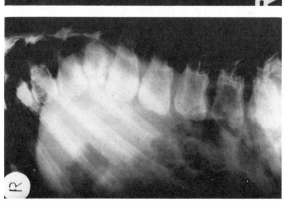

Fig. 9. An 8-yr-old. The vertebral changes are similar to those in Fig. 8. In addition, the body of L-1 is hypoplastic and dorsally displaced. There is mild hypoplasia of the basilar portions of the iliac bones. The hands are normal.

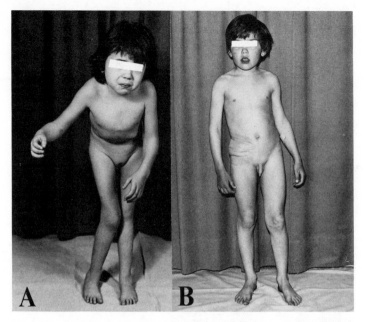

Fig. 10. A) A 9-yr-old, with β-galactosidase deficiency. Findings in this patient include coarse facial features, flexion contractures of the hips and spastic diplegia, defective visuomotor coordination, and mental retardation. First symptoms appeared at 13 months. Height 105 cm (below 3rd percentile). (For skeletal changes, see Fig. 8). B) An 8-yr-old, with β-galactosidase deficiency. Notice the coarse facial features. The patient is mentally retarded and suffers from extrapyramidal, mostly choreoathetoid movements. His visuomotor coordination is impaired. Height 127 cm (50th percentile) (For skeletal changes, see Fig. 9.)

artificial and natural substrates including glycoproteins, glycopeptides, glyco-saminoglycans, and G_{M1} ganglioside. A disturbance in the metabolism of the former substances probably relates to the mesenchymal changes and that of the ganglioside to the neurologic abnormalities. A mutation causing absent activity toward G_{M1} with preserved activity toward glycoproteins will result in a disease with severe neurologic but little skeletal involvement. Another mutation may impair the enzyme activity toward glycoproteins and glycosaminoglycans and have little effect on the enzyme's action on ganglioside. This mutation would result in a phenotype with marked skeletal abnormalities but with normal neuro-logic function.

Tissue-specific activity of β-galactosidase may be another factor causing vary-ing phenotypes. Cases have been described with low β-galactosidase activity in

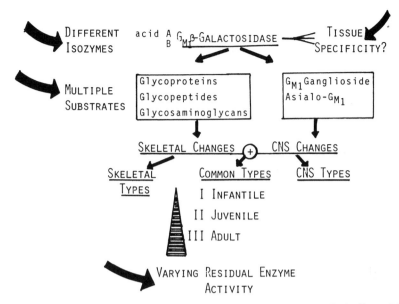

Fig. 11. Phenotypic variability of G_{M1} β-galactosidase deficiency. Hypothetically, variability can be expected from mutations which a) affect β-galactosidase differently in different tissues, b) affect only one of the two isozymes and/or their interaction, c) alter the catalytic properties of the enzyme toward some, but not all substrates, and d) alter the catalytic properties of the enzyme toward all substrates to different degrees (common types I, II, and III).

fibroblasts and leukocytes but high or normal activity in the kidney [29] or liver [27]. Finally, it should be remembered that there are different β-galactosidase isozymes with different catalytic activities. Possibly there are mutations that affect the relationship between these isozymes [37, 38].

In spite of the clinician's need for clear diagnostic criteria and classification systems, it seems prudent to heed Dr. O'Brien's advice on not to overclassify at present [34]. The distinction of three main types — infantile (I), juvenile (II), and adult (III) — is useful. One should, however, keep one's eyes open to the possibility of "atypical" cases. β-Galactosidase determinations are recommended whenever there is a dysostosis multiplex-like or spondyloepiphyseal dysplasia, and/or a neurodegenerative process associated with fine corneal opacities, vacuolized lymphocytes, or urinary excretion of keratan sulfate and galactose-containing glycoproteins.

REFERENCES

1. Hansemann D: Echte Nanosomie mit Demonstration eines Falles. Ber Klin Wochenschr 39:1209, 1902.
2. German J: Bloom's syndrome. Am J Hum Genet 21:196, 1969.
3. Grosse F, Gorlin J, Opitz JM: The Dubowitz syndrome. Z Kinderheilkd 110:175, 1971.
4. McKusick VA, Mahloudji MM, Abott MH, Lindenberg R, Kepas D: Seckel's bird-headed dwarfism. N Engl J Med 277:279, 1967.
5. Perheentupa J, Autio S, Leisti S, Raitta C, Tuuteri L: Mulibrey nanism, an autosomal recessive syndrome with pericardial constriction. Lancet 2:351, 1973.
6. Tympner K-D, Eichin F, Fendel H: Cockayne's Syndrom. Z Kinderheilkd 104: 298, 1968.
7. Beck GJ, van den Berg BJ: The relationship of the rate of intrauterine growth of low birthweight infants to later growth. J Pediatr 86:504, 1975.
8. Warkany J: "Congenital Malformations." Chicago: Year Book Medical Publishers, 1971.
9. Miller JD, McKusick VA, Malvaux P, Temtamy S, Salinas C: The 3-M syndrome: A heritable low birthweight syndrome. In Bergsma D (ed): "New Chromosomal and Malformations Syndromes." Miami: Symposia Specialists for The National Foundation—March of Dimes, BD:OAS XI(5):39—47, 1975.
10. Russell M, McDowell V, Sproles LT: The Russell-Silver syndrome. Am J Dis Child 126:794, 1973.
11. Spranger J, Opitz JM, Nourmand A: A new familial growth retardation syndrome: The "3-M syndrome." Eur J Pediatr 123:115, 1976.
12. Tanner JM, Lejanaga H, Cameron N: The natural history of the Silver-Russell syndrome: A longitudinal study of 39 cases. Pediatr Res 9:611, 1975.
13. Seckel HPG: "Bird-Headed Dwarfs." New York: Karger, 1960.
14. Bass HN, Smith LE, Sparkes RS, Gyepes MT: Case report 33. In Bergsma D (ed): "Syndrome Identification." White Plains: The National Foundation—March of Dimes, III(2):12, 1975.
15. Majewski F, Spranger J: Über eimen neuenTyp des primordialen Minderwuchses: der brachymele primordiale Minderwuchs. Monatsschr Kinderheilkd 124:499, 1976.
16. Jones KL, Smith DW: The fetal alcohol syndrome. Teratology 12:1, 1975.
17. Patterson JH: Presentation of a patient with leprechaunism. In Bergsma D (ed): Part IV. "Skeletal Dysplasias." New York: The National Foundation—March of Dimes, BD:OAS V(4):117—121, 1969.
18. David TJ: Unpublished observation. Bristol, 1976.
19. Wolcott CD, Rallison ML: Infancy-onset diabetes mellitus and multiple epiphyseal dysplasia. J Pediatr 80:292, 1972.
20. Spranger J: The metaphyseal dysplasias. In Bergsma D (ed): "Growth Problems and Clinical Advances." New York: Alan R Liss, Inc for The National Foundation—March of Dimes, BD:OAS XII(6):33, 1976.
21. Ammann A, Sutliff W, Millinchick E: Antibody-mediated immunodeficiency in short-limbed dwarfism. J Pediatr 84:200, 1974.
22. O'Brien JS: G_{M1} gangliosidosis. In Stanbury JS, Wyngaarden JB, Frederickson DS (eds): "The Metabolic Basis of Inherited Disease." 3rd Ed. New York: McGraw-Hill, 1972, p 639.
23. Goldberg MF, Cotlier E, Fichenscher LG, Kenyon K, Enat R, Borowsky SA: Macular cherry-red spot, corneal clouding, and β-galactosidase deficiency. Arch Intern Med 128:387, 1971.

24. Koster JF, Niermeijer F, Loonen MCB, Galjaard H: β-Galactosidase deficiency in an adult: A biochemical and somatic cell genetic study on a variant of G_{M1} gangliosidosis. Clin Genet 9:427, 1976.

25. Loonen MCB, van der Lugt L, Franke CL: Angiokeratoma corporis diffusum and lysosomal enzyme deficiency. Lancet 2:785, 1974.

26. Lowden JA, Callahan JW, Norman MG, Thain M, Prichard JS: Juvenila G_{M1} gangliosidosis. Arch Neurol 31:200, 1974.

27. Orii T, Minami R, Sukegawa K, Sato S, Tsugawa S, Horino K, Miura R, Nakao T: A new type of mucolipidosis with β-galactosidase deficiency and glycopeptiduria. Tohuku J Exp Med 107:303, 1972.

28. Pinsky L, Miller J, Shanfield B, Watters G, Wolfe LS: G_{M1} gangliosidosis in skin fibroblast culture: Enzymatic differences between types 1 and 2 and observation on a third variant. Am J Hum Genet 26:563, 1974.

29. Yamamoto A, Adachi S, Kawamura S, Takahashi M, Kitani T, Ohtori T, Shinji Y, Mishikawa M: Localized β-galactosidase deficiency. Arch Intern Med 134:627, 1974.

30. Wenger DA, Goodman SI, Myers GG: β-Galactosidase deficiency in young adults. Lancet 2:1319, 1974.

31. Feldges A, Müller HJ, Bühler E, Stalder G: G_{M1} Gangliosidosis. Helv Paediatr Acta 28:511, 1973.

32. Suzuki Y, Hayakawa T, Yazaki M, Hiratani Y: G_{M1} Gangliosidosis. A variant with high activity of hepatic neutral β-galactosidase. Eur J Pediatr 122:177, 1976.

33. Maroteaux P: Un nouveau type de mucopolysaccharidose avec athétose et élimination urinaire de kératan-sulfate. Nouv Presse Med 2:975, 1973.

34. O'Brien JS, Gugler E, Giedion A, Wiesmann U, Herschkowitz N, Meier C, Leroy J: Spondyloepiphyseal dysplasia, corneal clouding, normal intelligence, and acid β-galactosidase deficiency. Clin Genet 9:495, 1976.

35. O'Brien JS: Molecular genetics of G_{M1} β-galactosidase. Clin Genet 8:303, 1975.

36. Galjaard H, Hoogeveen A, Keijzer W, De Wit-Verbeek H, Reuser AJJ, Mae W-H, Robinson D: Genetic heterogeneity in G_{M1} – gangliosidosis. Nature 257:60, 1975.

37. Norden AGW, O'Brien JS: An electrophoretic variant of β-galactosidase with altered catalytic properties in a patient with G_{M1} gangliosidosis. Proc Nat Acad Sci 72:240, 1975.

38. Singer HS, Schafer IA: Clinical and enzymatic variations in G_{M1} generalized gangliosidosis. Am J Hum Genet 24:454, 1972.

The WT Syndrome—A "New" Autosomal Dominant Pleiotropic Trait of Radial/Ulnar Hypoplasia With High Risk of Bone Marrow Failure and/or Leukemia*

Claudette Hajaj Gonzalez, MD, Mary Virginia Durkin-Stamm, MS,
Nicholas F. Geimer, MD, Nasrollah T. Shahidi, MD,
Robert F. Schilling, MD, Francisco Rubira, MD, and John M. Opitz, MD

Since Fanconi [1] described a syndrome of refractory anemia and multiple congenital anomalies in 3 brothers in 1927, many other cases with that diagnosis have been published. In 1959, Garriga and Crosby [2] reviewed the literature to determine the incidence of leukemia and various anemias in other family members of patients with bone marrow hypoplasias, including those with Fanconi anemia. They defined Fanconi anemia as "progressive atrophy of the bone marrow associated with congenital abnormalities, or familial incidence of the disease, or both," and found reports of 66 such cases in 48 families. Developmental defects in nonanemic family members were found in 15 families, and leukemia in nonanemic family members was found in 4 families. There was no long-term follow-up in any of the families. They concluded that there existed a possible association between Fanconi anemia and leukemia and congenital defects in non-Fanconi syndrome family members, although their numbers were too small to prove such an association.

In 1964, Gmyrek and Syllm-Rapoport [3] reported the incidence of leukemia in the literature again to seek confirmation of the associations noted by Garriga

*Studies of Malformation Syndromes of Man: XLVI. Paper No. 2035 from the University of Wisconsin Genetics Laboratory. Supported by DHEW/PHS grant GM20130 from The National Institute of General Medical Sciences.

Birth Defects: Original Article Series, Volume XIII, Number 3B, pages 31–38
© 1977 The National Foundation

and Crosby [2]. They found such a high incidence of component manifestations in relatives that they concluded the Fanconi syndrome was an intermediate-dominant trait; neither set of authors seems to have considered the possibility that their patient material might represent a mixture of an autosomal recessive trait, namely, the Fanconi syndrome (with a rather high incidence of parental consanguinity) and one or more autosomal dominant traits with variable expressivity and no parental consanguinity.

We have studied 2 families with severe hypoplastic anemia, congenital anomalies, and leukemia and have defined an autosomal dominant trait — the WT syndrome — which we think has often been labeled "Fanconi syndrome" and which is responsible for the apparent occurrence of leukemia, other anemias, and congenital defects in "Fanconi syndrome" families in the literature.

CASE HISTORIES

The W Family (Fig. 1)

Patient II-2, male, was referred at 37 years with a 2-year history of chronic fatigue and a 5-week history of anemia, which did not respond to treatment with B_{12}, oral iron, or blood transfusions. No early history is available. He had unilateral cryptorchidism, abnormal elbows, 2 distal phalanges, and 2 nails on the left thumb, a hypoplastic, malformed right thumb without a metacarpal bone, shortness of both 5th fingers, pancytopenia, and marrow hypercellularity. No definite diagnosis was made.

Despite treatment with hydrocortisone, ACTH, B_{12}, pyridoxine, and some 125 units of blood, he died 3½ years after the onset of his disease, and at autopsy was

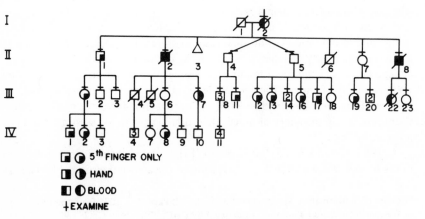

Fig. 1. The W Family.

found to have an increased amount of fat, but several good islands of hematopoiesis with a fair number of normoblasts in the marrow.

His brother, *II-8*, was also seen because of anemia. No early history is available on him, but he had been a regular blood donor until 27 years when mild anemia was detected; 6 months later he developed pancytopenia and severe anemia. Bone marrow showed hypocellularity with an M.E. ratio of 6.5:1. He received 15 transfusions as his only treatment in the 4 months before referral. Examination showed "short stubby fingers bilaterally," clinodactyly of the 5th fingers and some cutaneous syndactyly between the 4th and 5th fingers bilaterally, a small, nonfunctional thumb on the right, a simian crease on the right, and pancytopenia. In bone marrow he had very few nucleated cells which looked like lymphoid or histiocytic elements. There were no erythroid or granulocytic precursors. Despite treatment with testosterone, prednisone, and numerous blood transfusions, the patient died after 6 months. At autopsy he had a hypercellular marrow with 50% of the cells described as "large young cells" resembling lymphoid or tumor cells. The most likely diagnosis was acute stem cell leukemia.

His 11-year-old daughter, *III-22,* was referred for pancytopenia with a 1 month history of "flu," epistaxis, hematemesis, and treatment with 4 units of blood. Her previous history had been unremarkable. On admission she had acute lymphoblastic leukemia. The chromosomes were studied twice and showed a normal karyotype and no excess of breakage. She died 2 years later of CNS involvement. No congenital anomalies are recorded on the chart.

Her 71-year-old grandmother, *I-2,* was referred for a 10-year history of being easily bruised, a 3½ year history of pancytopenia, and more recently, epistaxis requiring transfusions. She had also received oral iron and hematinics. Physical examination purportedly showed no congenital anomalies. Laboratory studies showed a hypocellular bone marrow and she was discharged with the diagnosis of aplastic anemia (? aleukemic leukemia). A few weeks later a further evaluation revealed a hypercellular marrow with highly atypical cells. The diagnosis was acute (?) monocytic leukemia and she received several blood transfusions, prednisone, and oral iron. She died 1 month later, 3 years and 9 months after the onset of pancytopenia. No autopsy was performed.

The pedigree on the W Family is based on the family study done by Drs. Schilling and Geimer in 1962. Family members *II-1, III-11, III-12, III-13, III-16, III-17, IV-1,* and *IV-2* had clinodactyly of the 5th fingers, *III-1* and *IV-8* had short 5th fingers, *III-19* had short 5th fingers and clinodactyly, and *III-7* showed abnormal thumbs and clinodactyly of the 5th fingers. All the examined individuals (except *I-2*) had normal hematologic findings at that time.

The T Family (Fig. 2)

The propositus, *V-1,* was referred at 4 years for congenital hand anomalies. At 22 months he had had severe anemia (Hgb 5.5 g) requiring 2 transfusions after

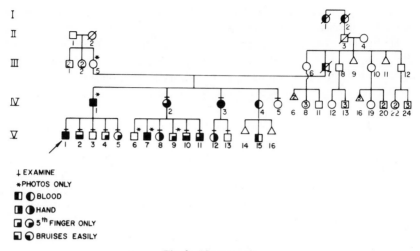

Fig. 2. The T Family.

unsuccessful oral iron treatment. His anemia improved spontaneously. Physical examination showed slight micrognathia, bilateral limitation of pronation and supination with posterior displacement of the head of the radius on the right, severe hypoplasia of both thumbs without motor function, and hypoplasia of both 5th fingers. Roentgenograms showed absence of the left 1st metacarpal, hypoplasia of the 1st phalanges more severe on the left, hypoplasia of both 5th metacarpals with partial fusion with the 4th metacarpal on the right, hypoplasia of the 5th phalanges, hypoplasia of the middle and distal phalanges of the index fingers, bilateral fusion of the greater and lesser multangulum and absence of the lunate. A pollicization was performed on the left side. His chromosomes showed a normal karyotype.

The patient's great-great-grandmother (I-2) and her sister (I-1) were both said to have been anemic; his great-grandfather (II-3) was reported normal and died of a heart attack at age 68; his grandfather (III–7) died at 51 years of acute myeloblastic leukemia – until 6 or 7 years he had been very sick with anemia. The patient's father (IV-1) has hypoplastic thumbs and short, clinodactylous 5th fingers, and was treated for anemia when 1 year old. He is now in good health. Three of the patient's sibs (V-2, V-4, and V-5) have clinodactyly and shortness of the 5th fingers. One of them (V-2) appears to bruise more easily than the others. One of the patient's paternal aunts (IV-2) has clinodactyly of the 5th fingers, ulnar deviation of right 3rd finger; she bruises easily. Her son (V-7) was slightly anemic after an attack of rheumatic fever at 5 years; he has hypoplastic thumbs and 5th fingers. His sister ((V-8) and brother (V-11) have never had any serious illnesses or anemias, but their hands are affected. Both show abnormal thumbs, proximally implanted with narrowed distal phalanges, hypoplastic thenar eminences, and short and clinodactylous 5th fingers. *V-10* and *V-11* bruise easily, and *V-9* and *V-10* have clinodactyly of the 5th fingers. *IV-3* was treated for severe bleeding tendencies requiring transfusions between ages 4 and 14 years. Her hands are severely affected: The left thumb is smaller than the right and both are camptodactylous, without creases, and show tapered distal phalanges. There is severe thenar hypoplasia bilaterally; both 5th fingers have small middle phalanges and show slight clinodactyly. She bruises easily. Her daughter (*V-12*) also has severely affected hands and she is the only one in the family with hyperpigmented skin. Her right anomalous thumb was excised at age 3 months and her left thumb is hypoplastic and camptodactylous. The 5th fingers are very short, clinodactylous, and show only one crease. Roentgenograms showed absence of the right 1st metacarpal, hypoplastic left 1st metacarpal and phalanges, and hypoplastic 5th middle and distal phalanges.

IV-4 was fine until 15 months when she had a severe ear infection treated with an unknown antibiotic. She developed a severe anemia. At the University of Wisconsin Hospitals her diagnosis was "a true blood dyscrasia" but its type was not established. She received multiple transfusions and at 6½ years she recovered spontaneously. There is no mention of congenital anomalies and we have not seen this woman. Her son *(V–15)* purportedly had "blood problems" as a baby.

We saw all of the W family members marked with a bar over their pedigree symbol. Most of those with "minor hand anomalies" were said to be normal by the family, as was the case of *IV–2* and *V–7*. Prolonged residence of both families in the same part of Wisconsin suggests that the W and T families may be branches of the same family.

Four families with probable WT syndrome have been reported in sufficient detail to be sure about the diagnosis; we think that many other reports of the "Fanconi syndrome" actually deal with the WT syndrome [4—6] but insufficient details preclude a firm conclusion.

REVIEW OF THE LITERATURE

McDonald and Goldschmidt [7] reported 3 children and their mother who had severe anemia in childhood. The oldest daughter was born with a supernumerary thumb. At age 6 years, she presented with anemia and was diagnosed as having aplastic anemia. ACTH, corticosteroids, vitamin B_{12}, folic acid, and iron as well as splenectomy were without benefit and she died at 10 years. Another daughter showed increasing pallor and tendency to bruise easily at 10 years; the diagnosis of hypoplastic anemia with neutropenia and thrombocytopenia was made. Her right thenar eminence was smaller than the left and she was incapable of abducting or extending the right thumb. A 7-year-old son had anemia, pancytopenia and abnormal thumbs. A follow-up paper by McDonald and Mibashan [8] indicated that these two children had recovered.

Coletta et al [9] described 2 brothers with "Fanconi anemia." The first one had mild syndactyly between the 2nd and 3rd toes bilaterally and at 6 months developed severe anemia and pancytopenia. He died 3 months later. The second brother had bilateral shortness and clinodactyly of the 5th fingers and shortness of the 1st metacarpals. He had always been anemic and at 6 years developed pancytopenia. He received intensive therapy; no follow-up is provided. The family history is remarkable: 3 sibs, the mother, 1 maternal aunt, and the maternal grandfather had finger anomalies.

Rodriguez-Vigil and coworkers [10] described a boy with a hypoplastic left thumb (amputated immediately after birth), a hypoplastic right thumb, bilateral clinodactyly of the 5th fingers, ulnar deviation of the 2nd fingers, and radial deviation of the hands bilaterally. At 7 years he developed severe anemia with thrombocytopenia and died at 9 years with the diagnosis of "Fanconi anemia." His mother had brachydactyly and severe clinodactyly of the 5th fingers and his sister had short 5th fingers.

The family described by Cowdell et al [11] was very similar to our W Family: Two brothers with hand and some other anomalies developed aplastic anemia and leukemia, respectively, as adults. The first one had brachydactyly and malformed thumbs. He presented a possible history of childhood anemia (at 11 years he had an unexplained hematemesis); at 22 years he developed pancytopenia and died one year later. The second brother had "failure to thrive" and at 7 years was given thyroid treatment. At 27 years he developed anemia with pancytopenia. He had long, thin fingers with very short 1st metacarpals and hypoplastic right thenar eminence, and possible monocytic leukemia. However, the marrow findings suggested a granulocytic origin of the leukemia. He died 4 weeks later.

Some hematologic findings in parents of patients with Fanconi anemia are reported in the literature. The mother of Crisalli and Sansone's patient [12] was found to have severe pancytopenia; neutropenia was reported in the patient's mother described by Genz [13]; anemia and leukopenia are mentioned in the mother of one of the patients reported by Sansone and Crisalli [14]. The mother of Gelli's patient [15] was a normal woman with slight peripheral pancytopenia and bone marrow hypoplasia.

CONCLUSIONS

We are continuing work on the delineation of the WT syndrome which we think is a dominantly inherited trait with variable expressivity, and virtually complete penetrance. Many relatives of our patients were said to have had no congenital anomalies, but several of the affected family members we examined also thought their hands were normal. Some of the hand anomalies are subtle and may include ulnar deviation of the 1st or 3rd fingers, shortness, clinodactyly and/or camptodactyly usually of the 5th fingers, and unusual tapering of the thumb with or without thenar hypoplasia. The significance of these was not appreciated until the more severe hand anomalies were found in the family.

We considered slight shortness and clinodactyly of the 5th fingers to be coincidental minor anomalies if there were no other hand anomalies present. We do not know if either or both is a sign of the WT syndrome. The same is true of "easy bruising." The people so coded were compared with their sibs. Information about bruising was not solicited but was mentioned by family members. Both *I-1* in the W Family and *IV-3* in the T Family gave a history of easy bruising for several years before the development of severe hematologic disease. Only time will tell if the people so coded in these 2 pedigrees do, in fact, have the WT syndrome. The various childhood anemias of these individuals were often treated, but always improved spontaneously.

The genetic aspects of this syndrome are important. If our hypothesis is true, relatives of Fanconi syndrome patients may not be at an increased risk of leukemia. Families with "adult" Fanconi syndrome, or Fanconi anemia associated with leukemia or congenital anomalies in non-Fanconi syndrome family members, or Fanconi anemia which resolves in childhood may represent the WT syndrome. In all such cases, all family members should be carefully examined and counseled regarding dominant inheritance. As far as we know to date, patients with the WT syndrome do not have shortness of stature, microcephaly, MR, eye anomalies, other major visceral anomalies, or extensive pigmentation, and results show they do not have increased chromosome breakage. In this connection it is important that such studies always be done blindly; some reports of increased breakage may, in fact, be invalid observations.

SUMMARY

We report 2 families with an autosomal dominant syndrome of limb and hematologic abnormalities.

The W Family was ascertained through AW, a 13-year-old girl, who was purportedly born without congenital anomalies and who was normal until 11½ years when she developed acute lymphoblastic leukemia. She died 2 years later with CNS involvement. Her chromosomes, studied in the first weeks after diagnosis of the disease, were apparently normal. Her father had clinodactyly of both 5th fingers and was found to have panmyelocytopenia refractory to all treatment at 26 years. He died within a year of the onset of his anemia. This man's oldest brother was born with congenital malformations of the elbows and the hands and was healthy until 38 years when he was also found to have an "idopathic anemia" and panmyelocytopenia which was refractory to treatment except for transfusions; he died at age 42 years. Both men were initially thought to have the Fanconi anemia syndrome. Their mother died at 71 years of leukemia.

DT, the propositus of the second family, was noted to have malformations of both hands at birth. At 21 months he had anemia for which he received transfusions. Family history reveals that several people on the paternal side have severe hand anomalies and a history of childhood anemia. The paternal grandfather died at age 51 of acute monocytic leukemia.

Barring genetic heterogeneity, we think that the trait in the W and T families is the same. It is a pleiotropic autosomal dominant mutant which affects radial and ulnar development of the upper limbs and is associated with a relatively high risk of transient or permanent bone marrow arrest with or without leukemia. We propose the hypothesis that apparently increased risk of leukemia to Fanconi heterozygotes actually represents admixture with the WT syndrome and that Fanconi heterozygotes may not have an increased risk of leukemia.

REFERENCES

1. Fanconi G: Familiäre, infantile perniziosaartige anämie. Jb Kinderheilkd 117:257–280, 1927.
2. Garriga S, Crosby WH: The incidence of leukemia in families of patients with hypoplasia of the marrow. Blood 14:1008–1014, 1959.
3. Gmyrek D, Syllm-Rapoport I: Zur Fanconi-anaemie: Analyse von 129 beschriebenen Fällen. Z Kinderheilkd 91:297–337, 1964.
4. Özer F: Fanconi panmyelopathy. In Bergsma D (ed): Part XVI "Urinary System and Others." Baltimore: Williams & Wilkins for The National Foundation–March of Dimes, BD:OAS X (4) 174, 1974.
5. Gutierrez M, Diaz L, Quesada J, Fainstein V, Gonzalez R: Anemia de Fanconi. Informe de un caso. Rev Invest Clin 25:189–198, 1973.
6. Rohr K: Familial panmyelophthisis: Fanconi syndrome in adults. Blood 4:130–141, 1949.
7. McDonald R, Goldschmidt B: Pancytopenia with congenital defects (Fanconi's anaemia). Arch Dis Child 35:367–372, 1960.
8. McDonald R, Mibashan RS: Prolonged remission in Fanconi-type anemia. Helv Paediatr Acta 6:566–576, 1968.
9. Coletta A, Esposito C, Palomby L: Aspetti clinico-ematologici ed interpretazioni patogenetiche della pancitopenia ipoplastica congenita con malformazioni multiple tipo Fanconi. Pediatria (Napoli) 69:7–28, 1961.
10. Rodriguez-Vigil E, Sanchez-Badia JL, Felipe-Lagunilla L, Gonzalez-Garcia E, Jimenez-Pindado F, Fernandez I, Hevia M: Pancitopenia constitucional con malformaciones congénitas. Enfermedad de Fanconi. Rev Esp Pediatr 19:397–414, 1963.
11. Cowdell RH, Phizackerley PJR, Pyke DA: Constitutional anemia (Fanconi's syndrome) and leukemia in two brothers. Blood 10:788–801, 1955.
12. Crisalli M, Sansone G: Constitutional infantile panmyelopathy with multiple malformations ("Fanconi anemia"). First Italian report. Helv Paediatr Acta 3:299–308, 1952.
13. Genz, H: Klinische Beobachtungen und Untersuchungen bei einem Fall von Fanconianämie. Arch Kinderheilkd 145:237–242, 1952.
14. Sansone G, Crisalli M: L'anemia di Fanconi. Rassegna sintetica e contributo clinico. Minerva Pediatr 5:971–987, 1953.
15. Gelli G: Pancitopenia ipoplastica familiare tipo Fanconi (anemia di Fanconi). Minerva Pediatr 11:1225–1232, 1959.

Autosomal Dominant Maxillofacial Dysostosis

Michael Melnick, DDS, and John R. Eastman, DDS

Autosomal dominant maxillofacial dysostosis (maxillofacialis syndrome) is a little-known variant of the first and second arch syndromes. The physical findings in these patients include: 1) anterior-posterior shortening of the maxilla occasionally resulting in a relative mandibular prognathism; 2) antimongoloid slanting of the palpebral fissures; 3) minor malformations of the auricles; 4) severely delayed onset of speech with poor vocabulary development and poorly connected discourse; 5) nonfluent and inarticulate speech including prolongations, hesitations, and vowel and consonant substitutions, omissions, and distortions. There is phenotypic variability in the cases thus far investigated and this may be evidence for heterogeneity.

In addition to the cases in this report, to our knowledge there are only two fairly well-documented cases in the literature. In 1932, Villaret and Desoilles [1] described a "primary familial hypoplasia of the maxilla." In three generations of this family there were three persons (paternal grandfather, father, and son) who had a congenital hypoplasia of the maxilla with a relatively mild mandibular prognathism. The maxilla was shortened in the lateral and anterior-posterior dimensions. There were no other malformations, but the father is described as having poor intellectual development. From the pedigree the inheritance was clearly autosomal dominant with complete penetrance. In 1960, Peters and Hövels [2] described a father and son with a mid-face deficiency that included maxillary hypoplasia, antimongoloid slant of the palpebral fissures, a narrow parrot-beaked nose, a flattened "frontonasal angle," open bite, and aplasia of the lobule of the ear. The radiographs demonstrated a maxillary hypoplasia along with a shortness of the cranial base. The authors reported a relative tongue hyper-

Birth Defects: Original Article Series, Volume XIII, Number 3B, pages 39–44
© 1977 The National Foundation

plasia (owing to the maxillary hypoplasia) that they assumed to be responsible
for what they termed the "mechanically retarded speech." The occurrence in this
family was also consistent with an autosomal dominant inheritance.

CASE REPORTS

Proband A is a 4-year-old white male with a height of 109.86 cm (75th%),
a weight of 18.6 kg (75th%) and a head circumference of 52 cm (+ 1 SD). He is the
product of a full-term uncomplicated pregnancy and delivery and weighed 3.2 kg
at birth. He sat at 7 months, crawled at 13 months, and took his first step at 16
months, but he did not walk until 23 months. His speech had been greatly delayed
and he had not completed toilet training at the time of examination. The child
appeared well-proportioned and alert, and he reacted normally to the usual
stimuli. He was normocephalic and had significant malar hypoplasia and no
mandibular hypoplasia (Fig. 1). The sutures were closed and there was no
ridging. The posteriorly rotated ears were simple in architecture and short in
the vertical dimension with a hypoplastic lobule and lower helix. The external
auditory canals were patent but unusually small. There was antimongoloid slant
of the palpebral fissures, but there were no palpebral or iris colobomas. The
shape of the nose appeared to be within the limits of normal variation. He had

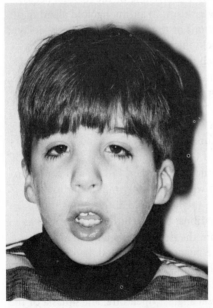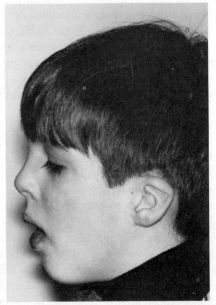

Fig. 1. Note the malar hypoplasia, antimongoloid slant of palpebral fissures, and the unusual
shaped and posteriorly rotated ears.

a somewhat constricted palate but dental development was essentially normal.

The skin, hands, feet, arms, and legs were all normal. There was hypertrichosis of the arms, legs, and back. The child had retarded speech development; he did not speak until 3 years. The mother stated that whole sentences were a recent development. He had a language age of 2.5–3 years, and conspicuous nonfluency and inarticulation. Single-word comprehension was measured at the 4th percentile for chronologic age. He could count to 3 but was unable to name colors and the Stanford-Binet Scale indicated a mental age in the 3–3.5 year range. Hearing acuity was normal.

The maxillary length (PNS-ANS = 43.7 mm) was reduced (Fig. 2) and malar hypoplasia was obvious (Fig. 1). The upper facial height and mandibular length (ramus and body) were within normal limits. The impression was clearly one of maxillary hypoplasia.

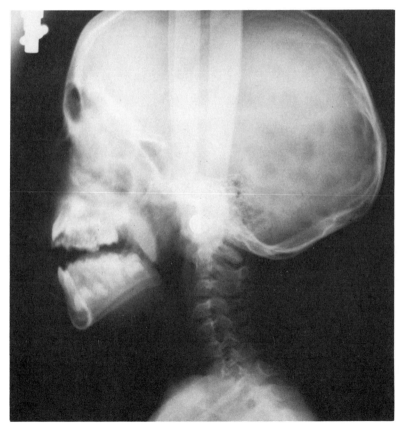

Fig. 2. Lateral cephalogram demonstrating maxillary hypoplasia.

The proband's mother (Fig. 3) is 35 years old, well-proportioned, alert and intelligent. Her speech, hearing, and comprehension were normal. She was normocephalic, had malar hypoplasia and apparent mild micrognathia. The ears, eyes, nose, skin, hair, and limbs were normal. She was also somewhat hirsute. Cephalometric analysis [3] revealed a flat and short cranial base (2 SD less than the mean for age) (Fig. 4). The maxillary length was 2 SD less than the mean for age but the upper facial height was normal. The body of the mandible was short (3 SD less than mean) and the gonial angle was obtuse (2.5 SD greater than mean). The ramus of the mandible and lower facial height were within normal limits. It should be noted that although the maxilla and mandible were short there was no relative flattening of the middle face (ANB angle 3°; normal: 2.6° ± 2.4°). Thus, the impression was one of a proportionate hypoplasia of the entire splanchnocranium — a situation somewhat different from that of her son but quite similar to that of the affected son in the report by Peters and Hövels [2].

The proband's father and brother were examined and found to be without abnormalities. The remainder of the family history was noncontributory.

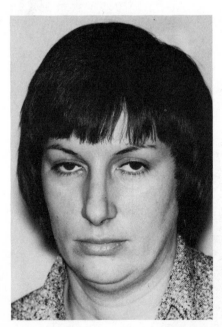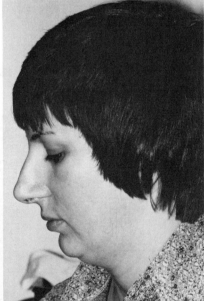

Fig. 3. Mother of proband.

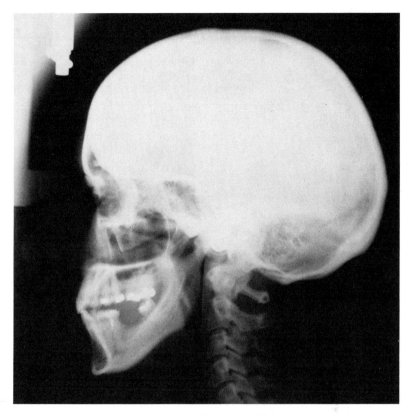

Fig. 4. Lateral cephalogram showing proportioned reduction of the entire splanchnocranium.

DISCUSSION

The differential diagnosis of maxillofacial dysostosis includes the other more common branchial arch syndromes (Table 1). On the basis of the small number of known cases, it appears that the minimal diagnostic criteria for this syndrome include maxillary hypoplasia and significantly retarded development of speech and language skills without marked IQ depression. Its differential diagnosis from mandibulofacial dysostosis is based primarily on a lack of severe mandibular hypoplasia and presence of retarded language development and inarticulation in the absence of deafness. The extent (if any) of mental subnormality remains unclear at this time.

The known cases of this syndrome represent autosomal dominant inheritance. Vertical transmission and male-to-male transmission have been observed.

TABLE I. Differential Diagnosis

Physical findings	Maxillo-facial dysostosis	Mandibulo-facial dysostosis	Hemifacial microsomia	Oculo-auriculo-vertebral dysplasia
Mandibular hypoplasia	±	−	+[a]	+[a]
Maxillary hypoplasia	+	+	+[a]	+[a]
Antimongoloid slant of the palpebral fissures	+	+	−	+
Eyelid coloboma	−	+ (Lower)	−	+ (Upper)
Malformation of auricles	+	+	+[a]	+[a]
External auditory canal defects	−	+	+	+
Conductive deafness	−	+	+[a]	+[a]
Scalp hair on lateral cheek	−	+	−	−
Retarded language development[b]	+	−	−	−
Speech inarticulation[b]	+	−	−	−
Vertebral anomalies	−	−	−	+

[a]Typically unilateral only
[b]In the absence of deafness

ACKNOWLEDGMENTS

This is publication #76-17 from the Department of Medical Genetics and was supported in part by the Indiana University Human Genetics Center PHS GM 21054, Individual NIH Postdoctoral Fellowship F22 DE 01274 and the Oral-Facial Genetics Institutional Grant DE 00007.

REFERENCES

1. Villaret M, Desoilles H: L'Hypoplasie primitive familiale du maxillaire supérieur. Ann Méd 32:378–381, 1932.
2. Peters A, Hövels O: Die Dysostosis maxillo-facialis, eine erbliche, typische Fehlbildung des 1. Visceralbogens. Z menschl Vererb u Konstit-Lehre 35:434–444, 1960.
3. Riolo ML, Moyers RE, McNamara JA, Hunter WS: "An Atlas Of Craniofacial Growth: Cephalometric Standards from the University School Growth Study, The University of Michigan." Ann Arbor: Center for Human Growth and Development, 1974.

Acrofacial Dysostosis With Growth and Mental Retardation in Three Males, One With Simultaneous Hermansky-Pudlak Syndrome

Thaddeus E. Kelly, MD, PhD, Richard J. Cooke, MB, BCh(Dubl), and Richard W. Kesler, MD

We report three males with a syndrome of short stature, mild acrofacial dysostosis, genitourinary anomalies and mild mental and growth retardation probably inherited as an autosomal recessive, or possibly X-linked, disorder. One of the three patients also had features of the Hermansky-Pudlak syndrome.

CASE REPORTS

Case 1 was the product of a term pregnancy to parents who were double first cousins. He had severe intrauterine growth retardation; at birth he weighed 1.9 kg, was 43 cm long, and was noted to have hypospadias, undescended testes, and unusual facies. Roentgenograms demonstrated maxillary and mandibular hypoplasia. Chromosomes were 46,XY. He had three normal older sibs.

At 13½ years (Fig. 1) he weighed 33.3 kg and was 137 cm tall (both < 3rd percentile). He had undergone successful repair of the hypospadias with orchidopexy and herniorrhaphy. He had a highly arched palate with a nasal voice tone. The palpebral fissures slanted downward. His arms showed limited supination with symphalangism of the thumbs and distal IP joints of the index fingers. He had a bilateral high-frequency hearing loss and a full-scale IQ of 58. An IVP was normal and skeletal x ray films were normal.

Case 2 was born after a term pregnancy to a 17-year-old primigravida and her 24-year-old husband. At birth he weighed 2.1 kg, was 47.5 cm long (intrauterine growth retardation), and was noted to have hypospadias with undescended testes. An IVP was normal and skull roentgenograms showed maxillary and mandibular hypoplasia. A partial duplication of the helix of the left ear was repaired. The

Birth Defects: Original Article Series, Volume XIII, Number 3B, pages 45–52
© 1977 The National Foundation

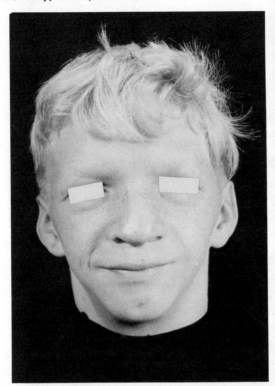
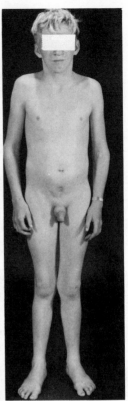
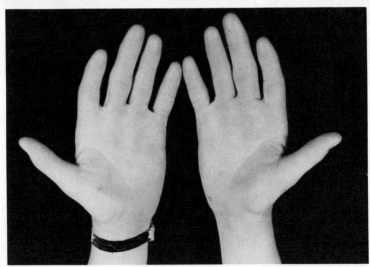

Fig. 1. *Case 1* at 13.5 years showing prominent brow, short stature, symphalangism of thumbs, and hypoplasia of distal IP flexion creases.

foster parents reported that his parents were cousins. One brother is included as *Case 3* and a third brother was normal (Fig. 2).

He was referred for evaluation of hypertension. At 15.5 years (Fig. 3) he was 158 cm tall, weighed 43 kg, and had a BP of 186/120. He had a prominent brow with downward-slanting palpebral fissures, flat malar eminences, a high, short palate with nasal speech. He demonstrated oculocutaneous albinism with minimal iris, hair, and skin pigmentation. He had symphalangism of the thumbs and distal IP joints of the index fingers. There was decreased flexion of the distal IP joints of the remaining fingers. Roentgenograms showed bilateral radioulnar synostosis. Femoral pulses were weak. He had a high-frequency hearing loss and a full-scale IQ of 52.

An aortogram revealed a partial obstruction of the aorta just superior to the renal arteries (Fig. 4). Plasma renin, cortisone, and electrolytes were normal. Complete blood count, platelet count, and bleeding and clotting times were normal. Platelet aggregation studies with ADP and epinephrine were abnormal. A bone marrow aspirate showed darkly pigmented macrophage inclusions. A peripheral lymphocyte culture revealed a normal 46,XY banded karyotype. However, compared to his brother, similarly affected with acrofacial dysostosis (*Case*

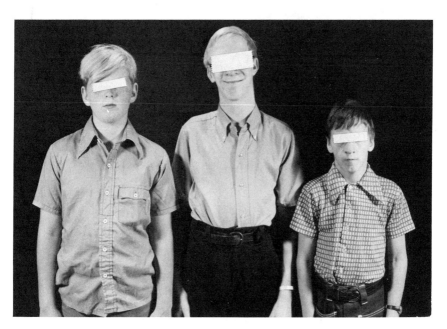

Fig. 2. Three brothers, left to right are 11 years, 15.5 years *(Case 2)* and 12 years 7 months *(Case 3)*.

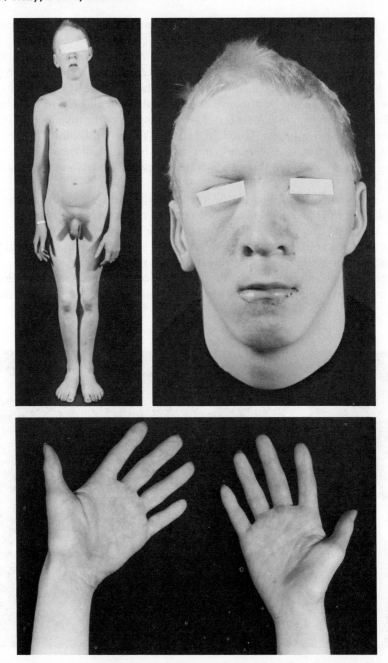

Fig. 3. *Case 2* at 15.5 years showed decreased pigmentation, short stature, symphalangism of thumbs with hypoplasia of distal IP flexion creases.

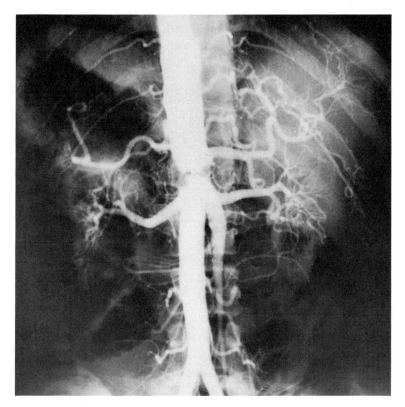

Fig. 4. Aortogram of *Case 2* with partial obstruction.

3) but no albinism and normal controls, there was a tenfold increase in spontaneous chromosomal aberrations.

At surgery the aortic obstruction was found to be secondary to plaque formation. A successful endarterectomy was carried out and postoperatively the patient has remained normotensive on no medication. Fresh platelets were available, but no unusual bleeding was encountered. Lipoproteins, cholesterol, and triglycerides were normal.

Case 3 was the younger brother of *Case 2*. At birth after a term pregnancy, he weighed 2.0 kg and was 45 cm long (intrauterine growth retardation). Glandular hypospadias and a unilateral undescended testis were noted.

At 12 years and 7 months he was 137 cm tall and weighed 27.5 kg (Fig. 5). The face was remarkably similar to that of *Cases 1* and *2* and distinctly different from that of the third brother. There was decreased extension and supination at the

elbows with unilateral radioulnar synostosis seen radiographically. There was symphalangism of the thumbs and index fingers with decreased distal flexion of the
remaining fingers. He had a high-frequency hearing loss and a full-scale IQ of 50.
A banded karyotype was 46,XY.

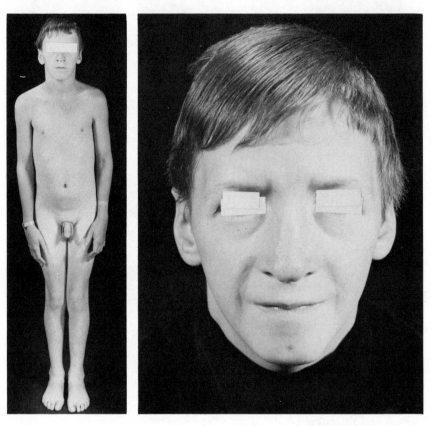

Fig. 5. *Case 3* at 12 years and 7 months with similar facies and short stature.

DISCUSSION

Malformation syndromes inherited as single-gene disorders are descriptively
delineated and classified. Significant intrafamilial variability results in wide phenotypic limits and in phenotypic overlap among syndromes. The limb manifestations of the thrombocytopenia absent radius syndrome and Fanconi anemia
syndrome are examples.

The combination of mild mandibulofacial dysostosis with preaxial, upper limb anomalies has been designated the Nager syndrome [1, 2]. This disorder is demonstrated in Figure 6 by a 2-year-old male. The limb anomalies consisted of bilateral radioulnar synostosis and hypoplasia of the thumbs. A more severe form may be represented by two unrelated newborns we have observed with absent thumbs, radioulnar humeral synostosis and severe mandibulofacial hypoplasia resulting in respiratory obstruction and right heart failure.

The three males described here demonstrate preaxial limb anomalies with mild mandibulofacial hypoplasia. In addition, they show intrauterine growth retardation with later short stature, mental retardation, and genitourinary anomalies. These cases do not fit the current definition of the Nager syndrome. If they represent a new entity, we favor autosomal recessive inheritance based on the consanguinity and the simultaneous occurrence of an additional autosomal recessive disorder, the Hermansky-Pudlak syndrome, in one of the three. With three affected males, X-linked inheritance remains possible.

The diagnosis of the Hermansky-Pudlak syndrome [3] in *Case 2* was based on the oculocutaneous albinism, abnormal platelet aggregation studies, and pigmented

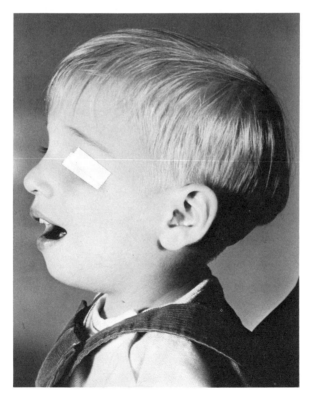

Fig. 6. Mandibulofacial dysostosis in 2-year-old male with the Nager syndrome.

macrophages on bone marrow aspirate. The pseudocoarctation seen in this patient is considered to represent a complication of the Hermansky-Pudlak syndrome. Bednar et al [4] reported the autopsy findings on one of the original patients with this disorder. They found thickening of adventitial tissue in the vicinity of large vessels and alteration of vessel structure by the accumulation of pigmento-phages in different layers of the vessels, which split and frayed the connective tissue fibers in the vessel wall.

Maurer et al [5] studied platelet function in albinism and reported three sibs with features of the Hermansky-Pudlak syndrome. They incidentally noted increased chromosome breakage in the sibs. Our patient demonstrated a tenfold increase in spontaneous chromosome aberrations over controls. This finding may further aid in the diagnosis of the Hermansky-Pudlak syndrome.

REFERENCES

1. Temtamy S, McKusick VA: Synopsis of hand malformations with particular emphasis on genetic factors. In Bergsma D (ed): Part III. "Limb Malformations." New York: The National Foundation—March of Dimes, BD:OAS V(3):125, 1969.
2. Bowen P, Harley F: Mandibulofacial dysostosis with limb malformations (Nager's acrofacial dysostosis). In Bergsma D (ed): "Limb Malformations." Miami: Symposia Specialists for The National Foundation—March of Dimes, BD:OAS X(5):109, 1974.
3. Hermansky F, Pudlak P: Albinism associated with hemorrhagic diathesis and unusual pigmented reticular cells in the bone marrow; report of two cases with histochemical studies. Blood 14:162—169, 1959.
4. Bednar B, Hermansky F, Lojda Z: Vascular pseudohemophilia associated with ceroid pigmentophagia in albinos. Am J Pathol 45:283—291, 1964.
5. Maurer HM, Buckingham S, McGiloray E, Spielvogel A, Wolff JA: Prolonged bleeding time, abnormal binding of platelet serotonin (5-HT), absent platelet "dark body," defective platelet factor 3 activation, bone marrow inclusions and chromosomal breaks in albinism. Proceedings of the Twelfth Congress, International Society of Hematology, New York: 1968, p 198. (Abstract.)

Acrocephalopolydactylous Dysplasia*

B. Rafael Elejalde, MD, Cesar Giraldo, MD, Raul Jimenez, DDS, and
Enid F. Gilbert, MD

CLINICAL AND GENEALOGIC STUDIES

At the birth of the propositus mother and father were 32 and 40 years old, respectively, living and well. They were first cousins; 3 of the mother's 13 pregnancies ended in spontaneous abortions before the third month of gestation (Fig. 1). Eight female and two male children were born after uneventful gestations; the last two, a male and female, respectively, had the new syndrome; the first eight were normal in all respects. A father's brother married a first cousin and had eight children, one of whom purportedly was affected with the same syndrome.

Patient 1

Spontaneous labor began at 34 weeks. Examination at 19 hr showed a cyanotic and edematous fetal leg in the vagina and a giant fetus in a breech position on the roentgenogram. The male fetus was delivered by cesarean section and died after minutes. The weight of the fetus and placenta was 7,500 and 3,500 gm, respectively. The infant was 51 cm long; circumference measurements included: occipitofrontal head circumference (OFC) 39 cm, chest 38 cm, lower limbs 13 cm, and upper limbs 12 cm. Examination showed: a swollen, almost globular body with virtual absence of neck, short limbs, apparently swollen face distorting the mouth and making the nose almost invisible and both palpebral fissures appearing as deep slits (Fig. 2). The fetus also had absence of the anterior fontanel,

*Studies of Malformation Syndromes of Man: XLIV. Contributed, in part, as paper No. 2037 from the University of Wisconsin Genetics Laboratory. Supported in part by DHEW/PHS grant GM20130-02 from the National Institute of General Medical Sciences.

Birth Defects: Original Article Series, Volume XIII, Number 3B, pages 53–67
© 1977 The National Foundation

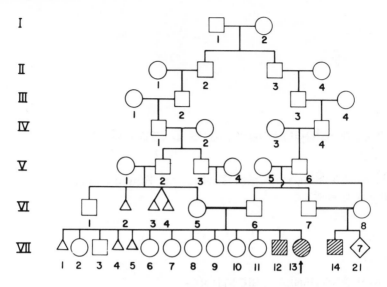

Fig. 1. Pedigree; *VII-12* is *Patient 1*; *VII-13* is *Patient 2*.

malformed auricles, mongoloid slanting of palpebral fissures, hypoplastic simple nose, micrognathia, redundant tissues of neck, voluminous thorax and abdomen, small omphalocele containing peritoneum and bowel, normal male genitalia with descended testes, and exceedingly thick skin which could not be picked up in folds and was called "edematous" by the obstetrician.

Autopsy showed complete closure of all cranial sutures and fontanels, a 0.5 cm thickness of the cranial base and a normal pituitary. The vertebras and limb skeleton were described as without malformation. The CNS was "immature" and showed vascular congestion and subarachnoid and perivascular hemorrhage. The skin was thick and fetal fat was present in the pericardium. Except for a patent ductus arteriosus, the heart and great vessels were unremarkable; however, in smaller vessels a remarkable perivascular proliferation of nerve fibers was found. The lungs weighed 10 gm each, did not contain air, and showed atelectasis. The liver was enlarged (370 gm), but the spleen was grossly normal; the peritoneal cavity contained 1,500 ml of ascitic fluid. The gastrointestinal tract was normal but the kidneys were enlarged: both measured 14 × 3 × 9 cm, weighed 45 gm, retained fetal lobulations, and had a thick fibrous capsule and multiple cysts as in a sponge kidney (Fig. 3) without showing clear-cut differentiation between cortex and medulla. Endocrine glands were normal.

Fig. 2. *Patient 1.*

Fig. 3. Kidney of *Patient 1.*

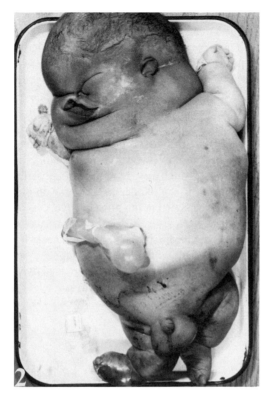

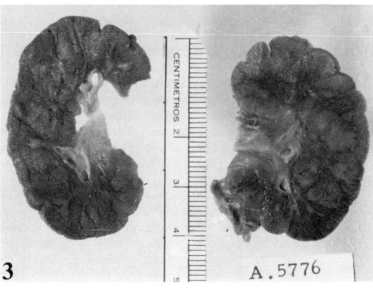

Microscopic studies confirmed subarachnoid hemorrhage, perivascular proliferation of nerve fibers in myocardium, thymus, pancreas, kidney, intestine
(primarily the colon near the cecum), and the capsule of the spleen; the spleen
also showed acute passive congestion. Lymph nodes showed lymphoid hyperplasia but the thymus was otherwise normal. "Epithelial spongiosis" with perivascular proliferation of nerve fibers was conspicuous in the tongue. An extraordinary amount of connective tissue was seen in the wall of the gut, primarily
in the colon. Interlobular fibrosis and foci of extramedullary hematopoiesis were
seen in the pancreas. Sections of renal tissue showed multiple glomerular cysts
with proliferation of epithelium of Bowman capsule, multiple cavities lined with
cuboid epithelium, unusual redundancy in number of collecting tubules, connective tissue proliferation around the tubules and underneath the renal capsule.
Multiple nerve fibers were also seen in the prostate.

In summary, this 34-week fetus had gigantism with an extraordinary excess
of subcutaneous connective tissue especially of trunk, neck, face and to a lesser
degree, of limbs, universal craniosynostosis, small omphalocele, malformed
auricles, relative micrognathia, hepatomegaly, cystic renal dysplasia, proliferation
of perivascular nerve fibers in myocardium, spleen, kidney, thymus, prostate,
pancreas, adrenal, tongue, and colon. No laboratory or cytogenetic examinations
were performed.

Patient 2

Three months after the birth of *Patient 1* his mother conceived again and
had a normal pregnancy until 34 weeks when an abdominal roentgenogram demonstrated a monstrous fetus who died 15 min after delivery by cesarean section
(Fig. 4). This female fetus weighed 4,300 gm and had a similar excess of subcutaneous connective tissue of trunk, neck, and limbs, apparent shortness of
limbs, in this case with hexadactyly of both upper limbs, an acrocephalic skull
with flat, tall forehead, flat supraorbital ridges, apparent hypertelorism with
thick, complete epicanthic folds, flat bridge and tip of nose with reduced length
of nasal septum, prominent capillary hemangiomatosis of forehead, glabella, and
nose, abnormally formed and distorted auricles, stiffness of the limbs, normal
female external genitalia, and small omphalocele. The length was only 39 cm,
OFC 35 cm, chest circumference 46 cm, abdominal circumference 49 cm, arm
circumference 15.5 cm, and thigh circumference 17.5 cm (measured at the
middle third of the limb).

Autopsy demonstrated an essentially normal skeleton, but the following
features were observed: complete fusion of all cranial bones and fontanels, a
grossly normal CNS for age, a thick dermis (3.5 cm), normally formed thoracic
organs with pulmonary hypoplasia, superior displacement of the diaphragm due
to hepatomegaly, small omphalocele containing intestine with otherwise normally appearing gastrointestinal tract, enlargement of kidneys with multiple

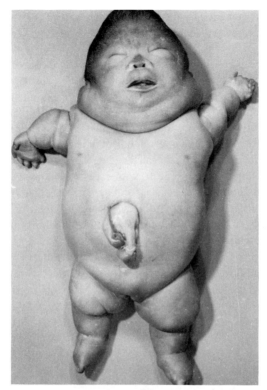

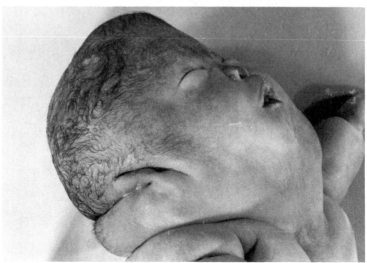

Fig. 4. *Patient 2.*

cysts but clear corticomedullary differentiation; the rest of the viscera and endocrine glands appeared grossly normal, but a supernumerary spleen was found near the kidney.

Microscopic studies showed pulmonary atelectasis, extraordinary proliferation of perivascular nerve fibers in myocardium (Fig. 5), capsule of spleen, pancreas (Fig. 6), tongue, intestine, prostate, and elsewhere extramedullary hematopoiesis in liver and pancreas, proliferation of biliary canaliculi and connective tissue (Fig. 7), greatly increased amounts of connective tissue, or fibrosis, of intestinal wall (primarily in the colon), surrounding dilated pancreatic ducts and ductules and lobules of submucosa of gall bladder (Fig. 8); Potter type 2 or multicystic dysplastic kidney changes (Fig. 9) with excessive connective tissue surrounding tubules and under the capsule, focal hemorrhage, dilatation of tubules, paucity of glomeruli, multiple glomerular cysts with proliferation of epithelium of Bowman capsule, and many other cavities lined with cuboid epithelium. The muscular fibers were distorted and had abnormal rounded, triangular shapes; proliferation of connective tissue was found in the skeletal muscle (Fig. 10). The epiphyseal lines had fewer cells than normal, but the other layers of bone formation were normal (Fig. 11). Lymph nodes showed lymphoid hyperplasia, but thymus, cardiac structures, uterus, adrenals, and CNS were within normal limits.

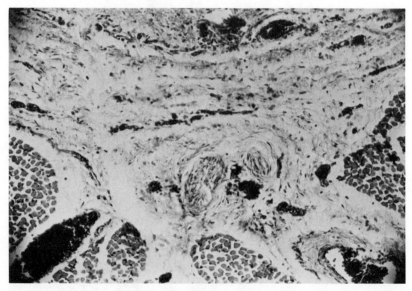

Fig. 5. Proliferation of nerve fibers and connective tissue in the myocardium. Hematoxylin-eosin stain X65.

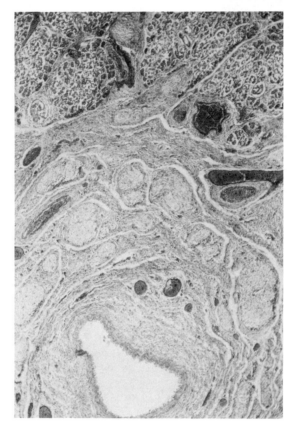

Fig. 6. Pancreas—striking proliferation of connective tissue and of nerve fibers around the arteries. Hematoxylin-eosin stain X65.

There was excessive connective tissue in the submucosa of the gall bladder, and the vaginal wall was greatly thickened by excessive connective tissue.

Routine, autoradiographic, and G-banding studies of chromosomes of lymphocytes and fibroblasts showed an apparently normal 46,XX chromosome constitution.

CELL KINETIC STUDIES

Trypsinized fibroblasts from *Patient 2* and a normal "control" fetus were planted in Leighton tubes containing medium 199 supplemented with 20% fetal

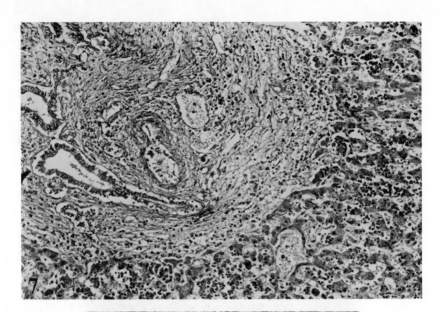

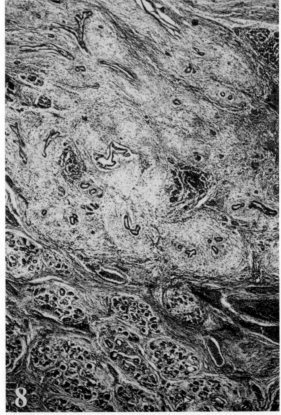

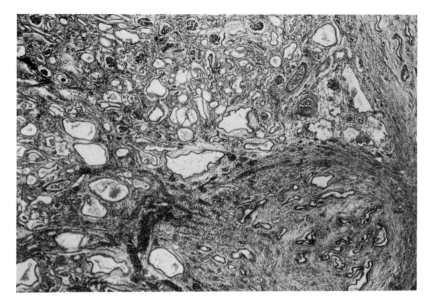

Fig. 9. Kidneys—paucity of glomeruli, multicystic dysplasia, and marked proliferation of connective tissue surrounding the tubuli. Hematoxylin-eosin stain X65.

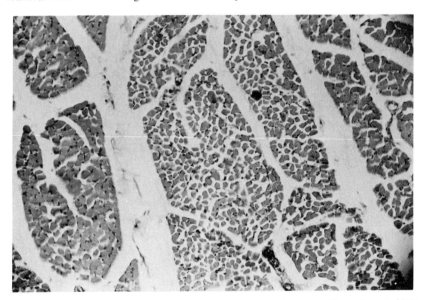

Fig. 10. Muscle—note abnormal shape of the muscular fibers. Hematoxylin-eosin stain X65.

Fig. 7. Liver—proliferation of connective tissue and of bile canaliculi. Hematoxylin-eosin stain X65.

Fig. 8. Pancreas—marked connective tissue proliferation within the acini and dilatation of the pancreatic ducts. Hematoxylin-eosin stain X65.

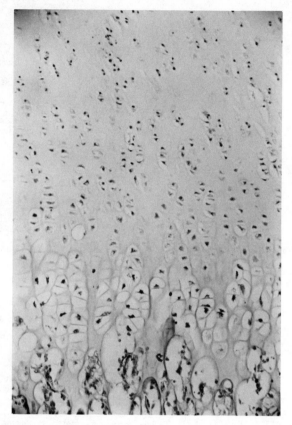

Fig. 11. Epiphyseal cartilage—paucity of cells in growth line. Hematoxylin-eosin stain X65.

calf serum. To each tube was added tritiated thymidine, 0.2 μCi/ml (thymidine 6-T(n), Batch 25 TRK 61, 10,000 mCi/m mol from the Radiochemical Centre, Amersham, England). Every hour, for 28 hours, mitoses were arrested in each of two tubes with Colcemid; after staining with synthetic orcein (Gurr, London), the slides were covered with autoradiographic emulsion (Agfa, Gevaert Scientia), exposed for 14 days, developed in D19B, and fixed.

A 5 ml sample of bone marrow was obtained at autopsy; each 0.5 ml was suspended in 4.5 ml of medium and cultured in the same way as a peripheral lymphocyte sample. Several 3 ml samples of the culture were arrested every hour for 16 hours and studied autoradiographically as before. The mitotic index was established for the patient's fibroblast and bone marrow cells and for control fibroblasts; the results are graphed in Figure 12.

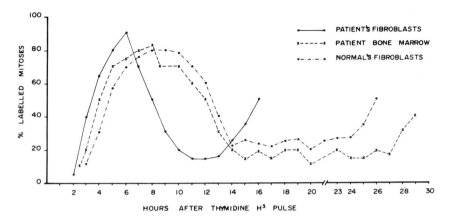

Fig. 12. Results of studies of DNA synthesis in patient's marrow cells and fibroblasts, and in normal fibroblasts.

This figure shows that the patient's bone marrow cells behaved essentially like normal fibroblasts, taking approximately 27 hours to complete the cell cycle; however, the patient's fibroblasts completed the whole cycle in 16-18 hours which is only about 63% of the normal time.

DISCUSSION

According to other literature, the condition discussed in this paper is a previously undescribed causal genesis syndrome due to the homozygous state of a rare autosomal recessive mutation [1].

Phenotypic analysis leads to the conclusion that this disorder is a true multiple congenital anomaly/dysplasia (ie, malformation/dysplasia) syndrome [2]. The predominating feature appears to be the dysplasia which is clearly of early prenatal onset and which may, in fact, have been responsible for some or all of the malformations.

Based on only two incompletely studied patients, we should like to suggest the following phenotypic analysis of the syndrome (Table 1):

The Malformations

These include polydactyly (probably postaxial) of the upper limbs; minor facial anomalies as described and illustrated above, malformation of the external ears (difficult to evaluate in *Patient 2* because of the severe distortion and involvement with the subcutaneous connective tissue hyperplasia); complete, premature, and atypical craniosynostosis was responsible for the congenital absence of fontanels and acrocephaly in *Patient 2* which was not associated with any of the syndactylous digital anomalies of the type seen in the other acrocephalosyndactyly syndromes; the small omphalocele seen in both patients is an anomaly of incomplete development and may be related to the hepatomegaly and/or connective tissue dysplasia of the abdominal wall surrounding the umbilical ring; the patent ductus arteriosus of *Patient 1* probably is a secondary reflection of pulmonary abnormality rather than a primary malformation.

Growth/Size Disturbances

These are probably all secondary manifestations of the dysplasia, though a length of 51 cm for a 34-week-old fetus suggests true acceleration of long bone length and/or vertebral height, even correcting for swelling of soles and increased thickness of scalp over the vertex. Though its size appeared normal in both cases, brain growth may have been slowed by the universal craniosynostosis; the increased occipitofrontal head circumference (OFC) (39 and 35 cm, respectively) for gestational age (34 weeks) may reflect increased thickness of scalp. The limbs appeared short; however, since no postmortem skeletal survey was obtained it was not possible to determine if this was true shortness or apparent shortness due to the peripheral extension of truncal tissue. Enlargement of gall bladder and ureteromegaly may represent a defect of innervation; vaginomegaly seems to have been due to an excess of connective tissue in the wall of that organ. The reason for the hepatomegaly remains unknown (excessive proliferation of biliary canaliculi?); it seems reasonable to conclude that the enlargement of that organ was at least in part responsible for the elevation of the diaphragm.

Pulmonary hypoplasia and atelectasis may represent effects of diaphragmatic elevation, altered chest wall dynamics (rigidity due to "armor plate effect"), an unknown component of oligohydramnios and/or limitation of swallowing, and complications of the cesarean section.

Stiffness of limbs probably represents limitation of fetal movement due to "armor plate" effect of thick skin and subcutaneous tissue; the same is probably true of the mild-to-moderate micrognathia.

Dysplasia

Three aspects of dysplasia command greatest attention in this syndrome: a) Renal dysplasia; b) Excess connective tissue virtually everywhere except in the CNS and concentrated most prominently subcutaneously, in the media of vessels, the walls of viscera, and interstitially in such organs as the pancreas, kidney, and wall of vagina; and c) Perivascular proliferation of nerve fibers in many viscera, primarily spleen, thymus, colon, heart and adrenal glands. There may be a close pathogenetic relationship between a and b; in any event, both seem to represent a hyperplastic mesodermal dysplasia whereas c seems to represent a hyperplastic ectodermal dysplasia. Hence, it seems most appropriate to think of the dysplasia in this syndrome as a hyperproliferative mesectodermal dysplasia. We think that the clear difference in the proliferative kinetics of the fibroblasts of *Patient 2* explains the enormous excess of connective tissue which is seen in this syndrome.

SUMMARY

We recently studied a male and his female sib who were the last of 13 pregnancies which included three spontaneous abortions and eight normal children who were born to normal, but consanguineous (first cousin) parents. A brother of the father also married a first cousin and had eight children one of whom purportedly was affected with the same syndrome. The propositus and his sister had:

Congenital malformations. Hexadactyly of upper limbs in the female, complete atypical premature fusion of all cranial sutures with acrocephaly, multiple minor anomalies of face, nose, and auricles, strikingly abnormal appearance of the entire fetus with greatly increased thickness of skin causing distortion of face and auricles, apparent shortness of neck and limbs, swollen, globular body shape with protuberant abdomen, and small omphalocele containing viscera. The male had a PDA.

Abnormalities of size and growth. Both were delivered at 34 weeks gestational age by cesarean section due to giant size. The male weighed 7,500 gm (his placenta, 3,500 gm), his OFC was 39 cm, and he was 51 cm long; his affected sister weighed 4,300 gm and had an OFC of 35 cm. Increased OFC is probably due to greatly increased thickness of skin, abdominal protuberance and omphalocele to "ascites," and organomegaly (greatly increased size of kidneys, ureters, liver, and gall bladder, increased thickness of wall of gut). Brain size was normal or reduced, lungs were small and atelectatic.

Dysplasia was most noticeable as: a) excessive amounts of connective tissue virtually everywhere except in CNS, but most prominent in subcutaneous tissue and in walls of hollow viscera (eg gut, vagina), the media of vessels, and interstitially in pancreas and liver; (b) cystic dysplasia of kidneys (large sponge kidneys with fetal lobulations and thick fibrous capsules); and (c) perivascular proliferation of nerve fibers in many organs, primarily spleen, thymus, colon, heart, and adrenal glands. Both a and c may be considered as hyperplastic mesectodermal dysplasia. Cell kinetic studies showed that fibroblasts in this condition proliferate at twice the normal rate.

Recent studies on two infants with a complex malformation/dysplasia syndrome indicated these infants had a previously undescribed autosomal recessive condition.

TABLE 1. Clinical and Anatomic Characteristics of the Syndrome

Physical characteristics	Patient 1	Patient 2
Birthweight	7,500 gm	4,300 gm
Placental weight	3,500 gm	1,500 gm
Birth head circumference	51 cm	39 cm
Birth chest circumference	38 cm	46 cm
Birth abdominal circumference	43 cm	49 cm
Acrocephaly at birth	+	+
Absent fontanels at birth	+	+
Hypoplastic nose	+	+
Downward slanted palpebral fissure	+	+
Rudimentary auricles	+	+
Redundant thick neck skin	+	+
Short limbs	+	+
Omphalocele	+	+
Polydactyly	−	+
Epicanthic folds	+	+
Hypertelorism	+	+
Lung hypoplasia	+	+
Accessory spleen	−	+
Megabladder	+	+
Megavagina	−	+
Megaureter	+	+
Proliferation of perivascular nerve fibers in:		
Thymus	+	+
Spleen	+	+
Adrenal	+	−
Prostate	+	−
Pancreas	+	+
Kidney	+	+
Intestine	+	+
Myocardium	+	+
Tongue	+	+
Redundant connective tissue in:		
Skin	+	+
Intestine	+	+
Kidney	+	+
Pancreas	+	+
Spleen	+	+
Gall bladder	−	+
Suprarenal	+	+
Ureter	+	+
Bladder	+	+
Vagina	−	+

TABLE 1. Continued

Physical characteristics	Patient 1	Patient 2
Perilobular fibrosis	+	+
Pancreatic fibrosis	+	+
Sponge kidney	+	+
Cystic renal dysplasia	+	+
Interstitial hyperplastic connective tissue	+	+
Nephrogenesis	+	+
Cystic Bowman capsule	+	+
Abnormal glomerular capillaries	+	+
Collecting tube proliferation	+	+
Meconium peritonitis	−	+
Excessive proliferation of biliary canaliculi	+	+
Abnormal muscular fibers	+	+
Reduced cells in bone growth line	+	+
Hyperplastic lymph nodes	+	+

REFERENCES

1. Herrmann J, Opitz JM: Naming and nomenclature of syndromes. In Bergsma D (ed): "Malformation Syndromes." Miami: Symposia Specialists for The National Foundation–March of Dimes, BD:OAS X(7):69–86, 1974.

2. Gilbert EF, Herrmann J, Opitz JM: Dysplasia, malformations and neoplasia, especially with respect to the Wiedemann-Beckwith syndrome. In Nichols WW, Miller RW (eds). "Proceedings of Symposium Cell Proliferation and Differentiation." Camden: Institute Medical Research, 1975 (In press).

A Syndrome of Microcephaly, Mental Retardation, Unusual Facies, Cleft Palate, and Weight Deficiency

David D. Weaver, MD, and Christopher P. S. Williams, MD

This article reports a previously apparently undescribed syndrome of mental retardation, microcephaly, unusual facies and cleft palate in two sibs.

CLINICAL PRESENTATION

Patient 1

The pertinent features of the proband, now 32 years old, are presented in Tables 1 and 2, and Figures 1–8. His father and mother were 23 and 19 years old, respectively, at the time of his birth. The mother had severe nausea during the pregnancy and noted poor fetal movement. The patient was born at term with a normal birthweight and length, and a cleft palate (Table 1). The neonatal period was unremarkable. An unsuccessful operation to repair the cleft at 1 month left the patient with a large palatal defect. The operation was complicated by respiratory arrest and cyanosis. No further repairs have been attempted.

Growth and developmental retardation were noted early. He crawled at 18 months, sat at 2½ years, walked with support at 5 years, stood alone at 6 years, walked unassisted at 8 years, talked at 8–10 years, fed himself at 15 years and, finally and remarkably, attained toilet training at 31 years. At 24 years motor development was estimated at a 31-month level. A Peabody Picture Vocabulary Test at 31 years yielded a vocabulary level of 2¼ years. Speech reception threshold was 60 db in the right ear and 25 db in the left at that time.

His health has been excellent; he has had no other operations. At 22 years he was ill for 6 weeks with flu-like symptoms and fever. Subsequently his speech and motor coordination regressed.

Birth Defects: Original Article Series, Volume XIII, Number 3B, pages 69–84
© 1977 The National Foundation

TABLE 1. Measurements[a]

Birth	Proband	Sister	
Weight (kg)	2.9	3.12	
Length (cm)	53	54.5	
Age (years)	32.5	14	22
General			
Height (cm)	161	102	–
Weight (kg)	28	10.9	21.3
Occipitofrontal circum. (cm)	48	44	47
Arm span (cm)	149	–	–
Lower body segment (cm)	81	–	–
Upper/lower segment ratio	0.99	–	–
Height age (years)	14 4/12	4 2/12	–
Weight at height age (percentile)	3(−3[b])	3 (−2 1/2[b])	–
OFC	–5[b]	−4[b]	−5[c]
Craniofacial			
Ear length[d] (cm)	5.5		5.3
Inner canthal distance (cm)	2.8		2.9
Interpupillary distance (cm)	5.5		5.2
Palpebral distance (cm)	2.6		2.5
Outer orbital distance (cm)	10.1		10
Philtrum (cm)	1.5		1
Limbs			
Palm (cm)	9.4		7.5
Index finger (cm)	7.1		5.8

[a] Normal standards available from Smith [10].
[b] SD for height age.
[c] SD for chronologic age.
[d] Where bilateralness exists, only the right measurement is stated; the patients are essentially symmetric.

The proband is quite sociable, pleasant, and cooperative, and will sit placidly for extended periods without restlessness. At other times in an effort to communicate, he will interject incomprehensible nasal sounds into the conversation. He is able to follow simple verbal commands particularly if given with gestures. Although capable of some self-help skills, he does not understand money, numbers, or time. He has been noted to perspire heavily at times particularly over the forehead.

The patient has always been underweight in spite of a good appetite and adequate caloric intake. Measurements were first available at 17.5 years when he weighed 20.7 kg (45.5 lbs) and was 140.4 cm (55¼ in) tall. His weight at this time was well below the 3rd percentile (−4 SD) for his height age (10.5 years). A similar height/weight relationship (Table 1) was found at 32.5 years when his height was mildly reduced while his weight was equivalent to that of an 8-year-old.

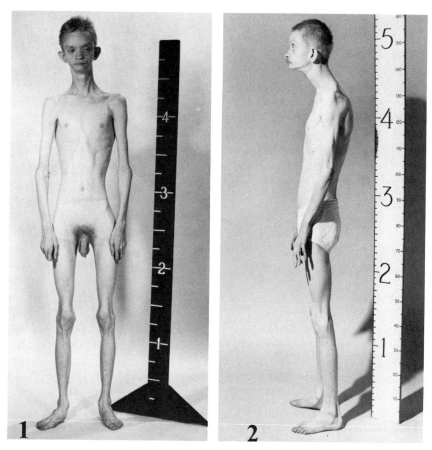

Fig. 1. Proband, age 24. Note the marked deficiency of muscle mass, the relatively normal height, and sexual development.

Fig. 2. Proband, age 32. Note the very thin limbs, the normal leg and trunk proportions. and positioning of the neck.

His small head and thin limbs give the proband a most unusual appearance (Fig. 1). The head circumference is 5 SD below the mean for the height age. At first glance he does not appear to be this microcephalic because his face is proportionally small and his neck is thin. He frequently holds his neck in an extended position (Figs. 2 and 4). Scalp and facial hair are thin, sparse and slow growing (he is shaved only once a week). The scalp hair pattern is normal. The eyes are deeply set, the ears are cupped, the jaw is micrognathic, and there is a right preauricular pit (Fig. 4). The tip of the nose is broad but not bifid (Fig. 3).

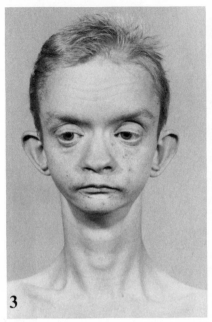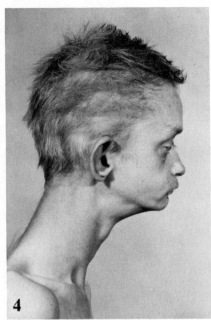

Fig. 3. Proband, age 24. Distinctive features include microcephaly, cupped ears, broad nose, small mouth with downturned corners, micrognathia and long thin neck. The microcephaly is difficult to appreciate in the presence of the diminutive face and thin neck.

Fig. 4. Proband, age 24. His diminished scalp and facial hair, midfacial hypoplasia, and slight prominence of the maxilla are notable.

The patient has severe gingivitis, extensive calculus formation, and marked discoloration of the teeth (Fig. 5). Some teeth are small and malformed while others are missing. These teeth are quite different from those seen in ectodermal dysplasia.

His muscle mass and strength are generally reduced, and the limbs and trunk are unusually thin. He has sustained clonus of both ankles, brisk patellar reflexes, a stiff-legged, wide-based, awkward gait, and poor balance. Body proportions are normal except for an alteration in the span-height ratio (Table 1). Dermatoglyphics are apparently normal.

A midsystolic murmur is thought to represent a functionally insignificant ventricular septal defect.

Major radiographic findings are listed in Table 2. In addition, skull films show orbital hypertelorism and a small calvarium. There is no indication of intracranial calcification. Generalized bone hypoplasia is present, particularly in the pelvic bones (Fig. 6). There is coxa valga and the ulnas and fibulas are short, hypoplastic, and show increased tubulation (Fig. 7). At 18 years his bone age was 11 years [1].

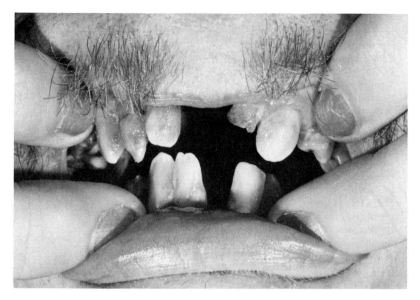

Fig. 5. Mouth of proband, age 32. Note the deficiency of anterior maxillary alveolar ridge with absence of teeth in this area, the fused, malformed and small teeth, and the poor oral hygiene.

Patient 2

The pertinent features of the proband's sister, now 22 years old, are presented in Tables 1 and 2, and Figures 9–13. She is the product of a pregnancy also characterized by severe nausea and poor fetal movement. In addition the mother had vaginal bleeding during the first trimester. Delivery was uncomplicated and at term. The birthweight and length were normal (Table 1). Except for a cleft of the soft palate she appeared to be normal in the immediate newborn period. Nevertheless, for the first 5 days, she had unexplained respiratory distress which resolved spontaneously.

Subsequently she has had marked developmental delay and deficiency of growth. She has never learned to roll over, sit up, stand, or speak, her developmental age now is estimated at 2 months. Her motor abilities have been hampered by the onset of myoclonic seizures and hemiparesis at 12 years resulting in the development of moderately severe flexion contractures, spasticity, and limited motion on the left side. The seizures were initially controlled by phenobarbital and later by diphenylhydantoin, the medication currently being used. An EEG at 13 years showed diminished activity over the right side but no localizing lesion or other abnormalities.

TABLE 2. Features

Performance	Proband	Sister
Mental retardation	+	+
Incomprehensible speech	+	+
Seizures and spasticity	−	+
Moderate hearing deficiency	+	?
Generalized		
Diminished subcutaneous tissue	+	+
Decreased muscle mass	+	+
Craniofacial		
Microcephaly	+	+
Prominent, hypoplastic ears	+	+
Preauricular pit	+	−
Midfacial hypoplasia	+	+
Deeply set eyes	+	±
Broad nose	+	−
Small downturned mouth	+	+
Malformed teeth	+	+
Cleft palate	+	+
Incisive maxillary papilla	+	+
Deficiency of anterior maxillary alveolar ridge	+	+
Limbs		
Extremely thin	+	+
Clinodactyly of fingers	+	+
Radiographic		
Generalized bone hypoplasia	+	+
Increased tubulation of bones	+	+
Reduced soft tissue layer	+	+
Tall but narrow vertebral bodies	+	+
Narrow pelvis with shallow acetabula	+	+
Delayed osseous maturation	+	+
Unusual down sloping ribs	+	+

+ = present, − = not present, ± = equivocal, ? = unknown

The patient has always had a poor appetite and has been difficult to feed. Before the onset of her seizures, she would take both liquid and pureed foods. Afterwards she has taken only liquids. Caloric intake has been adequate, however.

At 13 years she was institutionalized, initially in a state institution, but later in a nursing home near the family. They have continued to take an active interest in her and to participate in her care. During the last 8 years she has been in reasonably good health in spite of her condition.

Her facial appearance has changed considerably over the years. At 14 years (Figs. 9 and 10) her appearance was quite similar to that of her brother. At her

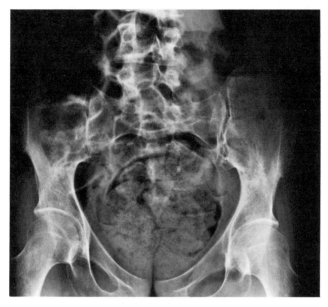

Fig. 6. Pelvis of the proband. Note the generalized bone hypoplasia and the shallow acetabula.

present age of 22 years, her facial features are coarser, the eyes are not as deeply set, the face is not as "pinched," and the jaw is prognathic, in comparison to her brother. In addition, she has kyphoscoliosis, a barrel-shaped chest, short neck, and strabismus, features not seen in the proband. She perspires normally.

She appears to be younger than her chronologic age. Behaviorally, she shows little interpersonal interaction with anyone. Her flexed left hand is frequently held in the right. Her feet are usually crossed and incessantly rubbed together. She will smile, grimace, and respond to painful stimuli.

She is microcephalic and has a normal scalp hair pattern. The orbital and mid-facial bones are hypoplastic. The ears, which are simple with a deficiency of the outer helices, are slightly posteriorly angulated but normal in position. There is poor oral hygiene with excessive dental calculus. Some teeth are oddly shaped; others are missing. Her cleft involves only the soft palate.

She shows generalized marked deficiency of muscle and subcutaneous tissue. A grade II/VI systolic murmur is detectable. Her breasts are small and axillary and pubic hair is scant. The dermatoglyphics, hand and feet creases, and general body hair distribution, are all normal.

The radiographic features show the same basic changes as found in her brother (Table 2). As calculated from the index of Greulich and Pyle [1] her osseous maturation was at the 6-month level when she was 7 years old. Her left hip is subluxed (Fig. 13). Orbital hypertelorism is not present.

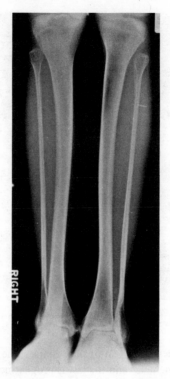

Fig. 7. Legs of the proband. Increased tubulation of the long bones and slight shortness of the proximal ends of the fibulas are obvious. Note the reduced soft tissue layer.

LABORATORY EVALUATION

No significant biochemical or chromosome abnormality has been found in either patient. Evaluation has included both Giemsa and quinacrine banding of the chromosomes, urine metabolic screening, complete blood count, multiple chemical screening of the serum (glucose, urea nitrogen, creatinine, electrolytes, uric acid, total protein, albumin, cholesterol, triglycerides, bilirubin, alkaline phosphatase, LDH, SGOT and CPK) and serum magnesium level. Serum calcium levels on two of three occasions were high or borderline high in the proband; ie 12.0 (age 24), 11.0 and 10.3 mg% (both age 32) (normal values 9–11 mg%). A serum calcium level in the sister at 21 years was normal.

FAMILY HISTORY

The pedigree is shown in Figure 14. The four other sibs and parents are normal and have average or above average intelligence. The facial appearances of the proband and his sister are unlike those of the rest of the family.

The other pregnancies were normal and quite different from those of these two. In all there were six miscarriages. They all occurred between two of the children. No explanation for their occurrence or for this unlikely distribution has been found. The parents are not consanguineous.

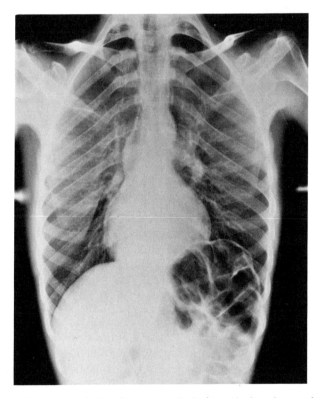

Fig. 8. Chest of the proband. The ribs are excessively down sloping, the muscles of the chest and shoulders are diminished, and the left hemidiaphragm is elevated.

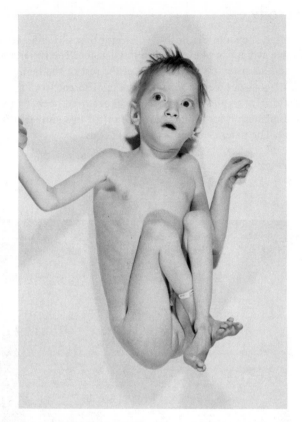

Fig. 9. The sister of the proband, age 14. She appears much younger than her chronologic age. Muscle deficiency is obvious. The clenched fist and flexed crossed legs are secondary to her hemiparesis and spasticity.

DISCUSSION

The condition of these two sibs seems to represent a previously undescribed dysmorphic syndrome. The primary features of this syndrome include moderate-to-severe mental retardation, microcephaly, weight deficiency, prominent ears, midfacial hypoplasia, cleft palate, clinodactyly of the fingers, delayed osseous maturation and generalized bony hypoplasia. The pattern of growth exhibited by these patients is characterized by postnatal growth deficiency of bone, muscle, subcutaneous fat and brain tissue. The height has remained relatively unaffected.

There are accurate measurements of body proportions only for the proband (Table 1). While the upper to lower segment ratio is normal, which indicates normal trunk and leg proportions, the span minus height value is −12 cm. For a normal adult male this value would be +5 cm.

Many of the radiographic findings could be explained on the basis of reduced weight-bearing and spasticity. Those findings associated with decreased weight-bearing would include increased tubularity of long bones, bone deficiency, particularly of the pelvis, but also, shallowness of the acetabula and increased height of the vertebral bodies. The excessive down sloping of the proband's rib cage most

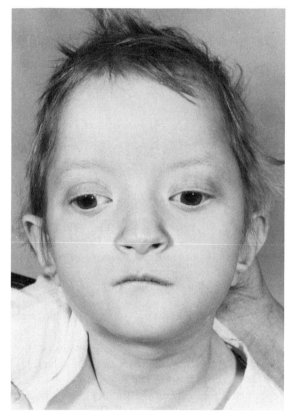

Fig. 10. The sister, age 14. Note the prominent ears, narrowness of the forehead, strabismus, telecanthus, and small mouth with downturned corners.

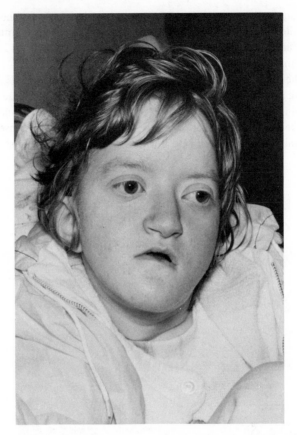

Fig. 11. The sister, age 21. The same basic facial features are present but they are of a coarser nature.

likely is from reduced strength. The sister's subluxed hip and the kyphoscoliosis are felt to be secondary manifestations of her hemiparesis and spasticity. The orbital hypertelorism seen in the skull film of the proband was not apparent clinically. In fact, his interpupillary distance is normal (Table 1).

No biochemical defect, chromosome aberration, teratogenic agent, or infection has been detected which would explain the etiology of this syndrome. It most likely represents an autosomal recessive trait, but the possibility that this is a segregating chromosome defect, inherited from one of the parents, is not completely ruled out.

The unique features of this syndrome allow it to be distinguished from previously described disorders that include mental retardation, microcephaly and weight deficiency as features. These conditions are the Seckel [2, 3], Cockayne [4, 5] and orocraniodigital syndromes [6], and progeria [7, 8].

The Marden-Walker syndrome [9] shares several characteristics in common with the condition described here but lacks microcephaly and mental retardation. Ectodermal dysplasia [10] is felt to be excluded by the presence of normal hair structure, nails and eccrine glands in the patients.

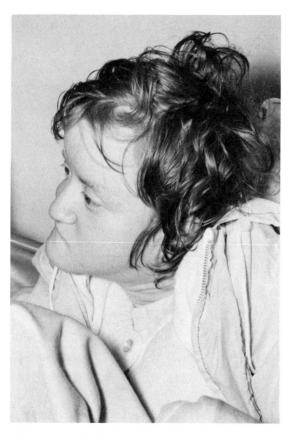

Fig. 12. The sister, age 21. Note the midfacial hypoplasia and prognathism.

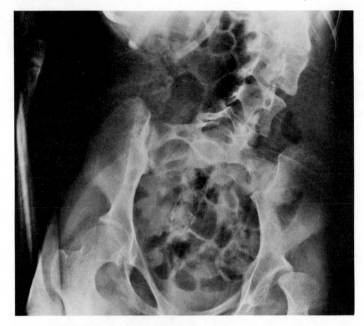

Fig. 13. Pelvis of the sister. The vertebral bodies are tall and the left femur is subluxed. Note the deficiency of bone of the pelvis and the scoliosis.

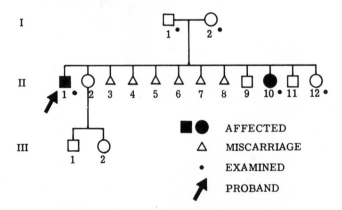

Fig. 14. Pedigree of immediate family. Ages as of May, 1976 are: *I-1*, 55; *I-11*, 51; *II-2*, 32; *II-9*, 24; *II-11*, 18; *II-12*, 14; *III-1*, 6; and *III-2*, 5. Miscarriages occurred before the third month for *II-4, 7* and *8;* at 4 months for *II-3, 6* and at 6 months for *II-5* all gestational ages.

SUMMARY

A brother and sister with a distinctive, apparently previously undescribed dysmorphic/mental retardation syndrome are presented. The major features of their condition include moderate-to-severe mental retardation, microcephaly, weight deficiency, prominent ears, midfacial hypoplasia, small mouth, cleft palate, clinodactyly of the fingers, delayed osseous maturation and generalized bone hypoplasia. Of these, the most prominent physical feature is the weight deficiency which is most likely the result of a decrease in muscle, bone, brain and subcutaneous tissue mass. No underlying biochemical defect, chromosome abnormality, environmental agent or infection has been found to explain this condition. An autosomal recessive mode of inheritance is suggested.

ACKNOWLEDGMENTS

The generous assistance of Drs. Al Hachman, Neal R. M. Buist, Eugene Blank and Edmund A. Franklen is graciously acknowledged. A special thanks goes to the mother of the patients. Without her cooperation and understanding, this report would not have been possible. Appreciation also goes to Drs. Doris H. Merritt, A. Donald Merrit, Robert D. Koler, M. E. Hodes, Joe C. Christian, and Rodney K. Beals, and to Ms. Lyn Tucker and Mrs. Suzanne Reynolds for their editorial assistance.

This work was done under NICHD Training Grant HD00165, University of Oregon Health Sciences and publication No. 76-44 from the Department of Medical Genetics, and supported in part by the Indiana University Human Genetics Center, PHS GM 21054.

REFERENCES

1. Greulich WW, Pyle SI: "Radiographic Atlas of Skeletal Development of the Hand and Wrist." Palto Alto, California: Stanford University Press, 1959.
2. McKusick VA, Mahloudji M, Abbott MH, Lindenberg R, Kepas D: Seckel's bird-head dwarfism. N Engl J Med 277:279–286, 1967.
3. Harper RG, Orti E, Baker RK: Bird-headed dwarfs (Seckel's syndrome), A familial pattern of development, dental, skeletal and central nervous system anomalies. J Pediatr 70:799–804, 1967.
4. Land VJ, Nogrady MD: Cockayne's syndrome. J Can Assoc Radiol 20:194–203, 1969.
5. MacDonald WB, Fitch KD, Lewis IC: Cockayne's syndrome – An heredo-familial disorder of growth and development. Pediatrics 25:997–1007, 1960.
6. Juberg RC, Hayward JR: A new familial syndrome of oral, cranial, and digital anomalies. J Pediatr 74:755–762, 1969.

7. DeBusk FL: The Hutchinson-Gilford progeria syndrome — Report of 4 cases and review of the literature. J Pediatr 80:697–724, 1972.
8. Gosh S, Varma KP: Progeria: Report of a case with review of the literature. Indian Pediatr 1:146, 1964.
9. Marden PM, Walker WA: A new generalized connective tissue syndrome. Am Dis Child 112:225–228, 1966.
10. Smith DW: "Recognizable Patterns of Human Malformation." 2nd Ed. Philadelphia: WB Saunders, 1976.

A New Variant of Ehlers-Danlos Syndrome: An Autosomal Dominant Disorder of Fragile Skin, Abnormal Scarring, and Generalized Periodontitis

Ray E. Stewart, DMD, MS, David W. Hollister, MD, and David L. Rimoin, MD, PhD

The Ehlers-Danlos (ED) syndrome is an inherited disorder of connective tissue which was originally described in 1682 by the Dutch surgeon, Job van Meekeran, [1] who reported a case which manifested "extraordinary dilatability of the skin." The eponym for this disease is derived from the names of two physicians who, over two centuries later, recognized the syndromic association of loose-jointedness, hyperelastic skin, subcutaneous hemorrhages, and subcutaneous tumors in several patients [2, 3].

The disorder was, for many years, thought to be a single entity, but has since been shown to exhibit extensive heterogeneity with at least seven distinct variants distinguishable by clinical and genetic criteria.

ED syndrome is one of several diseases classified generally as inherited disorders of connective tissue. The system most commonly used to classify the various forms of the syndrome was originally proposed by Beighton et al [4], and more recently modified by McKusick [5]. This system identifies seven distinct varieties of ED syndrome (Types I-VII), the characteristics of which are listed in Table 1. There have been numerous case reports in which the patients exhibited several of the physical findings of ED syndrome, but which do not fit well into any of the seven recognized types, suggesting the possibility of still more distinct diseases within this broad classification.

We have recently studied a family who appears to have a variant of the ED syndrome which does not fit into any of the seven currently recognized subtypes of this disease. The propositus had been referred from the UCLA School of Dentistry for evaluation to rule out a diagnosis of Marfan syndrome which had been considered due to the patient's asthenic habitus and marked arachnodactyly.

Birth Defects: Original Article Series, Volume XIII, Number 3B, pages 85–93
© 1977 The National Foundation

TABLE 1. Characteristics of Seven Variants of the Ehlers-Danlos Syndrome [6]

Types of Ehlers-Danlos syndrome	Skin hyperextensibility	Joint hypermobility	Skin fragility	Bruising
Severe (Type I)	Marked	Marked	Marked	Moderate
Mild (Type II)	Moderate	Moderate	Moderate	Moderate
Benign hypermobile (Type III)	Variable; usually marked	Marked	Minimal	Minimal
Ecchymotic (Type IV)	Minimal	Limited to digits	Marked	Marked
X-linked (Type V)	Marked	Limited to digits	Minimal	Minimal
Ocular variety (Type VI)	Marked	Marked	Minimal	Minimal
Procollagen peptidase deficiency (Type VII)	Moderate	Marked	Moderate	Moderate
New variant (? Type VIII)	Minimal	Moderate, limited to digits	Marked	Minimal

Medical History

The chief complaint was fragile skin and loose teeth. The medical history revealed that the propositus was the product of an uneventful pregnancy and delivery. He was born to a G2-P1-ABO female. Birthweight was approximately 3,405 gm. There were no significant problems during the neonatal or childhood periods, although the patient reported that he had always been tall and "skinny." He was aware of a problem of fragile, easily torn skin for as long as he could remember. This problem had been particularly prevalent on the anterior portions of his lower limbs.

Family History

The propositus, his father, and a male half-sib from a second marriage by the father, all had a history of fragile skin, peculiar scarring, and early loss of teeth due to severe periodontitis (Fig. 1). One of the father's parents may have been similarly affected. However, this cannot be substantiated because of inability to locate this part of the family.

Major complications	Inheritance	Basic defect
Musculoskeletal deformities common; varicose veins, prematurity due to ruptured	Autosomal dominant	Unknown
membranes	Autosomal dominant	Unknown
	Autosomal dominant	Unknown
Death from arterial rupture, aortic dissection, intestinal perforation; musculoskeletal abnormalities absent	Autosomal dominant	Type III collagen deficiency
Musculoskeletal disorders common	X-linked	Lysyloxidase deficiency
Fragility of cornea and sclera; musculoskeletal disorders	Autosomal recessive	Hydroxylysine deficiency
Marked short stature and multiple joint dislocations	Autosomal recessive	Procollagen peptidase deficiency
Fragility of skin, advanced generalized periodontitis	Autosomal dominant	Unknown

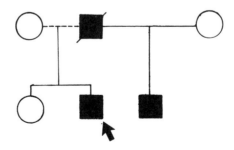

Fig. 1. Abbreviated pedigree of the family.

Physical Examination

This 21-year-old white male (Fig. 2). was 190.5 cm tall and weighed 54.5 kg. He had arachnodactyly (Fig. 3), numerous "cigarette-paper" scars (Fig. 4), and mild joint laxity, especially of the fingers (Fig. 5).Extensive scars over both shins consisted of very thin and translucent tissue (Fig. 6). These scars had resulted from mild blunt trauma, such as bumping the leg

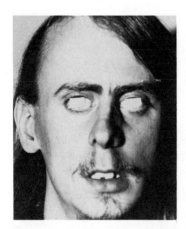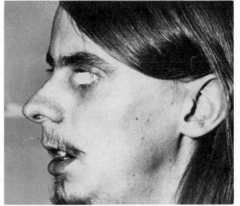

Fig. 2. Frontal and lateral facial photographs of the patient.

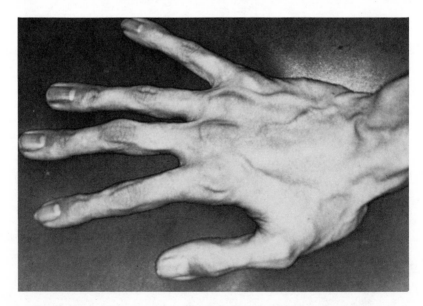

Fig. 3. Hand of the propositus with marked arachnodactyly and prominent viens.

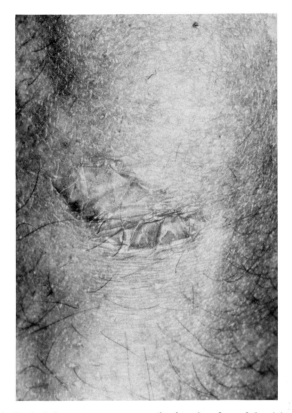

Fig. 4. Typical cigarette-paper scar on the dorsal surface of the right arm.

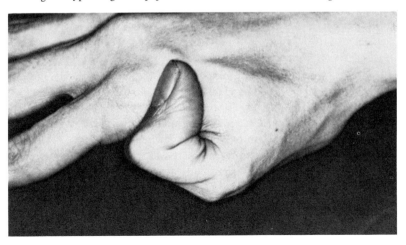

Fig. 5. Joint laxity — hyperextensibility of the patient's thumb.

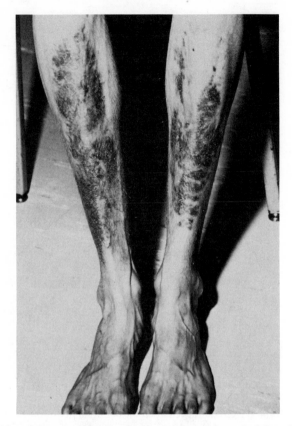

Fig. 6. The shins of the propositus showing the lesions which resulted from healing of skin tears following minor trauma to this region.

on a low table, which caused a rupture or tear of the skin and the development of a large hemotoma followed by gradual healing and replacement by the thin scar tissue.

Dental problems included extensive periodontal destruction, ie advanced generalized alveolar bone loss around all teeth, which had resulted in the premature loss of several permanent teeth. There was a propensity for the rapid and extensive formation of calculus, particularly around the gingival portions of posterior teeth. The periodontal pathology was very much like that seen in patients with Papillon-LeFevre syndrome of palmar and plantar hyperkeratosis with periodontitis (Fig. 7). The dental radiographs demonstrate the extensive bone loss seen around all permanent teeth (Fig. 8).

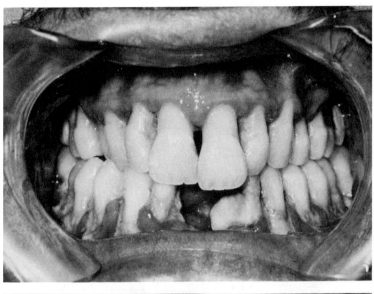
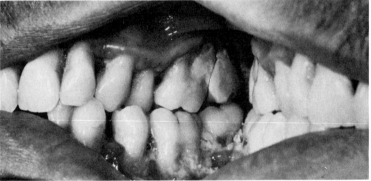

Fig. 7. Extensive periodontal disease and bone loss around all of the permanent teeth.

In the 4th edition of "Heritable Disorders of Connective Tissue," McKusick [7] mentions a condition which he termed "unique in his experience, and apparently in the literature as well," in which the wife of one of his colleagues and several of her relatives (her father, several aunts and uncles, and a cousin) shared an unusual array of anomalies. He described lesions on the shins similar to those observed in our patient, and reported slow-healing breaks in the skin following blunt trauma. The skin in his patient was not noticeably hyperextensible, nor

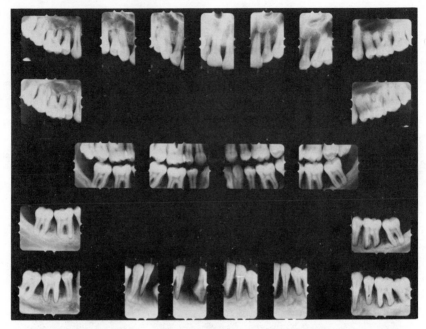

Fig. 8. Radiographs demonstrating nature and extent of alveolar bone loss around all permanent teeth.

were there any unusual cases of bruising. Joints were not hyperextensible. He reported that a second feature, "absorptive periodontitis," was syndromally related to the shin lesions. Several members of his family reportedly had cigarette-paper scars and redundant skin on the soles of the feet which are features that have been commonly reported in other types of Ehlers-Danlos syndrome.

Conclusions

It would appear that the family which we are reporting and the one mentioned by McKusick [7] have the same connective tissue disorder. In both families, the trait is most likely transmitted as an autosomal dominant. In both families, the affected individuals show advanced destructive periodontal disease at an early age in association with cigarette-paper scarring and unusual lesions on the shins which resemble necrobiosis diabeticorum lesions. This type of lesion has also been described in Type IV Ehlers-Danlos syndrome.

The propositus in our family had moderate joint laxity which was not noted in McKusick's family. In neither family was there marked hyperextensibility of the skin or marked bruisability (see Table 1).

The similarities of the observed anomalies in affected members of these families suggest that they represent yet another variant of the ED syndrome.

Since the most widely used system of classifying the various types of E D utilizes a numbering system (I—VII), we suggest that the syndrome we described be called Ehlers-Danlos Type VIII.

REFERENCES

1. van Meekeran JA: "De dilatabilitate extraordinaria cutis." Observations medicocliniques, Amsterdam, 1683, ch 32.
2. Danlos M: Un cas de cutis laxa avec tumeurs par contusion chronique des coudes et des genoux (xanthome juvenile pseudo-diabetique de M M Hallopeau et Mace de Lepinay). Bull Soc Franc Derm Syph 19:70, 1908.
3. Ehlers E: Cutis laxa, Neigung zu Haemorrhagien in der Haut, Lockerung mehrerer Artikulationen. Derm Zschr 8:173, 1901.
4. Beighton P, Price A, Lord J, Dickson E: Variants of the Ehlers-Danlos syndrome : Clinical, biochemical, haematological and chromosomal features of 100 patients. Ann Rheum Dis 28:228, 1969.
5. McKusick VA: Editorial: Multiple forms of the Ehlers-Danlos syndrome. Arch Surg 109:475, 1974.
6. Gorlin R: Heritable mucocutaneous disorders. In Stewart R, Prescott G (eds): "Oral Facial Genetics." St. Louis: CV Mosby, 1976.
7. McKusick VA: "Heritable Disorders of Connective Tissue." 4th Ed. St. Louis: CV Mosby, 1972.

Familial Fatal Neonatal Radiculoneuropathy

Richard C. Gilmartin, MD, W. Manford Gooch, III, MD,
Robert S. Wilroy, Jr, MD, and Emanuel Stadlan, MD

The study of diseases of the motor unit that affect the newborn is experiencing a period of rapid development. The poverty of our knowledge in this area is embodied in the noncommittal term, "the floppy infant" [1]. A hopeful sign is the recent appearance of case reports of children born with involvement of peripheral nerves [2, 3]. In general, the clinical and pathologic features in these cases are compared with those found in infantile spinal muscular atrophy [4, 5]. There is also an older body of literature describing cases whose symptoms began in infancy and early childhood, but who died at an older age [6]. In these cases pathologic studies document a lack of myelin, and to a lesser degree the failure to develop the normal population of axons. Peripheral nerves also show an increase in collagen fibers and are associated with a patchy denervation atrophy in skeletal muscle. In spite of growing interest in disorders that affect the motor unit in the young, almost no pathologic material is available in the first weeks of life [7].

This paper reports the clinical features in two infant cousins (*II-59* and *II-61* of Fig. 1) from a highly inbred Mennonite family who died with a similar congenital neuromuscular disorder. The autopsy findings in one of the infants is reported. An investigation of the pedigree (Fig. 1) uncovered four families that included the two cases reported in this paper and five additional relatives who all died prior to 3 months of age. Representatives from three generations of this family underwent a physical and clinical neurophysiologic examination and were found to be normal. The mothers of previously affected children have learned to expect a recurrence when they experienced decreased fetal movements associated with polyhydramnios.

Birth Defects: Original Article Series, Volume XIII, Number 3B, pages 95–101
© 1977 The National Foundation

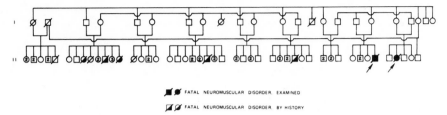

◼◗ FATAL NEUROMUSCULAR DISORDER, EXAMINED

◪◩ FATAL NEUROMUSCULAR DISORDER, BY HISTORY

Fig. 1. Pedigree of a family with a familial neonatal disease of the peripheral nerves.

CASE REPORTS

Case 1 (II-59) was born to a 25-year-old gr G6 P4 Ab1 white female following a 39 week pregnancy. Vaginal bleeding occurred in the first trimester and
polyhydramnios appeared in the latter half of the pregnancy. Fetal movements
were diminished throughout the pregnancy. A weak cry, inability to suck, areflexia, diminished muscle mass, and tachypnea characterized the immediate
neonatal period. The tachypnea and respiratory distress were associated with
absent diaphragmatic excursions and a pneumonitis unresponsive to antibiotics.
The child lay in an opisthotonic posture and appeared unresponsive to most
sensory stimuli. The Moro reflex was weak, and the root, suck, and grasp reflexes
were almost absent. Nevertheless, the child was able to twist his trunk and arms
when in distress.

The infant failed to gain weight and experienced a persistent watery diarrhea.
He was fed by a nasogastric tube, and at one time by peripheral hyperalimenta-
tion. A barium swallow demonstrated normal deglutition and peristaltic function
when a bolus was placed in the posterior oropharynx. Contrast material pooled in
the vallecula and pyriform sinus. The gastroesophageal valve was patulous with
gastric reflux to the midesophagus.

Neurophysiologic studies revealed unmeasurable sensory velocities, and slow
motor nerve conduction velocities. Sensory-motor cortical-evoked potentials
could not be elicited, and a neurogenic EMG pattern was more striking in the
distal musculature. The patient died at 35 days of age during one of many attacks
of bradycardia and cyanosis.

Case 2 (II-61) was born to a 20-year-old G2 P1 Ab0 white female of a pregnancy
complicated by decreased fetal movements and polyhydramnios. After a
3 hour labor, a 2,869 gm female was born. The cry was immediate but weak.
Even though resuscitation was unnecessary, her respirations remained shallow,
rapid, and ineffectual. She was unable to suck and was fed by nasogastric tube.
Oxygen was required intermittently because of cyanosis.

The course in the neonatal unit was characterized by shallow respirations,
tachypnea, weak cry, ineffectual suck, cyanotic episodes associated with seizure

activity and bradycardia, constant opisthotonic posturing, intractable diarrhea, and failure to gain weight. She was treated with phenobarbital, phenytoin, gentamicin, and nafcillin for pneumonitis and recurrent seizures.

The occipital frontal circumference was 36 cm. The patient had an opisthotonic posture, was restless, and had shallow respirations. Diaphragmatic excursions were imperceptible, and respiratory efforts were primarily by intercostal and accessory muscles. She was malnourished. Her limbs were tapering and almost devoid of muscle. Motor examination revealed hypotonia, diminished biceps, deep tendon reflexes, and absent triceps, knee and ankle tendon reflexes. The patient had facial diplegia with normal eye movements and no tongue fasciculations. Decreased suck, absent grasp, and very weak Moro reflexes characterized the transient responses of infancy.

Serum magnesium, calcium, SGOT, CPK, glucose, BUN, potassium, sodium, chloride, and osmolality were within normal limits. The serum bicarbonate tended to be low in the range of 14 meq/l. Spinal fluid examination revealed: glucose 76 mg/dl; protein 136 mg/dl; WBC 0/mm^3; RBC 49/mm^3. Chromosomal analysis of peripheral blood lymphocytes revealed an apparently normal karyotype (46, XX).

The patient was discharged three days prior to her death at 65 days of age.

PATHOLOGY

The postmortem examination on *Case 1* (*II-59*) revealed generalized, resolving pneumonitis. All portions of the gastrointestinal tract including its neural elements were normal. The brain weighed 560 gm and its gross appearance was normal. Central chromatolysis of scattered anterior horn cells of the spinal cord were present (Fig. 2). Similar changes were observed in the hypoglossal nucleus of the medulla, associated with a mild astrogliosis. In addition, older and more advanced changes were noted in other medullary nuclei, particularly the dorsal nucleus of the vagus nerve. Within this nucleus there was a marked decrease in the number of neurons and an associated reactive astrocytosis.

There was marked lack of myelin in the posterior columns of the spinal cord (Fig. 3). This was also seen in sections of the anterior and posterior roots and to a lesser degree in the sciatic and phrenic nerves. Sheath cell proliferation was noted within the sciatic nerve. There was also a reduced number of axons in the area of myelin loss. The loss of axonal elements were disproportionately less severe than the myelin loss.

Patchy neurogenic atrophy was seen in sections of the diaphragm. This was characterized by strikingly small muscle fiber groups intermixed with normal-appearing muscle fibers. Similar changes were noted in the iliopsoas and deep neck muscles.

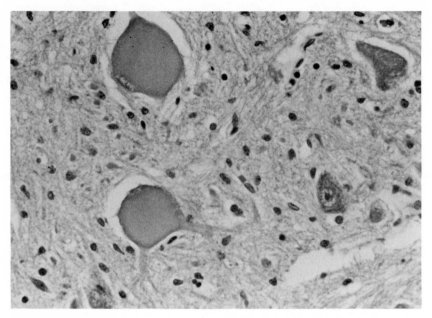

Fig. 2. Section of the anterior horn of the spinal cord showing central chromatolysis, swelling of the neurons, and rounding of the cell bodies. There is a minimal glial response.

DISCUSSION

Clinically, this entity fits into the poorly defined group of disorders described as the "floppy baby." However, its features, both clinical and pathologic, more closely resemble the case material described under the more specific heading of "infantile polyneuropathies" [2, 3].

When first seen, however, these children are most likely to be confused with progressive spinal muscular atrophy. However, there are striking clinical differences (Table 1). Polyhydramnios, distal muscle weakness, areflexia, diaphragmatic involvement, opisthotonic posturing, autonomic instability, and chronic diarrhea are not typically found in infantile spinal muscular atrophy. Pathologically, the involvement of the posterior columns, particularly the fasciculus gracilis, is uncommon. The lesion is commented upon by Marshall and Duchen [8], but in their series, affected children had a later onset of their symptoms and longer survival. Involvement of the sensory roots and posterior columns under the case heading of Werdnig-Hoffman disease was probably first described by Fredrick Batten [9]. However, in the rare cases subsequently described with posterior column involvement, the posterior rootlets were described as normal.

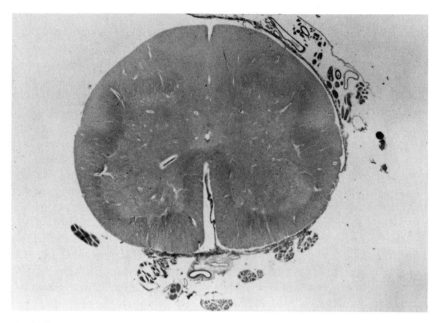

Fig. 3. Section of lumbar cord stained with Luxol fast blue to demonstrate myelin. There is a lack of myelin in the posterior columns, lateral spinothalamic tracts, anterior and posterior roots, and lateral corticospinal tracts. The posterior columns and rootlets are the first areas of the spinal cord to myelinate in fetal life.

TABLE I. Comparison of the Clinical Features in Werdnig-Hoffman Disease With the Reported Cases

	Neonatal polyradiculoneuropathy	Werdnig-Hoffman disease
Posture	opisthotonic	pithed frog
Weakness	distal	proximal
Respiration	accessory muscles of respiration	diaphragmatic
Pectus excavatum	present	present
Polyhydramnios	present	absent
Fetal movement	reduced	reduced
Diarrhea	present	absent
Nerve conduction	slowed	normal
EMG	neurogenic	neurogenic

The recent literature has described cases of early childhood polyneuropathy that simulate infantile spinal muscular atrophy. In these cases summarized by Goebel et al [2], the involved anterior and posterior roots have shown rounded islands of glial fibrils. These lesions have lead Chou and Fakadej [10] to propose that strangulation of anterior nerve roots by glial fibers is one of the causes of the loss of corresponding anterior horn cell motor neurons. This was not seen in our case.

Lack of myelin in the posterior roots, peripheral nerves, and posterior columns is apparently greater than the axonal loss. Some myelin loss would be expected secondary to axonal degeneration of both the central and peripheral nervous system. The observed quantitative dissociation between relative axonal preservation and myelin loss suggests that the myelin loss is a secondary phenomenon or that there is a primary arrest in the development of myelin. Biochemical studies may be able to define the pathophysiology of the myelin deficit.

There is good correlation between the pathology and most of the clinical features. The distal weakness, atrophy of limb musculature, and patterns of denervation can be correlated with the pattern of loss of motor neurons observed primarily in the cervical and lumbar regions. The diaphragmatic involvement is purely neurogenic and is associated with the changes seen in the peripheral nervous system (phrenic nerve).

The opisthotonic posturing could be viewed as reflecting the relative preservation of proximal muscle group function, particularly when compared with the almost total absence of distal motor function. Polyhydramnios in the absence of maternal factors, high gastrointestinal tract obstruction, or craniofacial anomalies suggests an early intrauterine onset of a neurogenic swallowing dysfunction [11]. This is supported by the more chronic and extensive degenerative changes observed in the vagal and hypoglossal nuclei. There is nothing in the pathologic study, however, to explain the diarrhea.

Apparently, there are various clinical entities presenting in the first weeks of life as "floppy infants" that are an expression of defective structure and function of the peripheral nerves. This report presents the clinical and pathologic findings on one apparently recessively inherited disorder that is uniformly fatal in the first months of life. A better clinical and pathologic delineation of the defects is necessary to better understand a metabolic and toxic disorder that interferes with normal myelination. Hopefully, this report will stimulate a search for autopsy confirmation and pathophysiologic explanations of clinical changes observed in neonates with diseases of their motor units.

REFERENCES

1. Dubowitz V: "The Floppy Infant." Clinics in Developmental Medicine, No 31. London: Heinemann Medical, 1969.

2. Goebel HH, Zeman W, DeMyer W: Peripheral motor and sensory neuropathy of early childhood simulating Werdnig-Hoffman disease. Neuropaediatrie 7(2):182–195, 1976.
3. Karch SB, Urich H: Infantile polyneuropathy with defective myelination: An autopsy study. Dev Med Child Neurol 17:504–511, 1975.
4. Byers RK, Banker BQ: Infantile muscular atrophy. Arch Neurol 5:140–164, 1961.
5. Greenfield JG, Stern RO: The anatomic identity of the Werdnig-Hoffman and Oppenheim forms of infantile muscular atrophy. Brain 50:652–686, 1927.
6. Tasker W, Chutorian AM: Chronic polyneuritis of childhood. J Pediatr 74:699, 1969.
7. Gilles FH: Myelination in the neonatal brain. Hum Pathol 7(3):244–248, 1976.
8. Marshall A, Duchen LW: Sensory system involvement in infantile spinal muscular atrophy. J Neurol Sci 26:349–350, 1975.
9. Batten FE: Progressive spinal muscular atrophy of infants and young children. Brain 433–463.
10. Chou SM, Fakadej AV: Ultrastructure of chromatolytic motorneurons and anterior spinal roots in a case of Werdnig-Hoffman disease. J Neuropathol Exp Neurol 30: 368–379, 1971.
11. Abramovich DR: In "Amniotic Fluid." Fairweather DVI, Eskes TK (eds). Amsterdam: Excerpta Medica 1973, pp 38–47.

The Pallister Mosaic Syndrome*

Philip D. Pallister, MD, Lorraine F. Meisner, PhD, B. Rafael Elejalde, MD,
Uta Francke, MD, Jürgen Herrmann, MD, Jürgen Spranger, MD
William Tiddy, DDS, Stanley L. Inhorn, MD, and John M. Opitz, MD

True multiple congenital anomaly/mental retardation (MCA/MR) syndromes have been divided into four groups [1]: 1) Those presumably caused by chromosome abnormalities, 2) those representing "known," nonchromosomal syndromes; 3) the idiopathic, sporadic cases, and 4) the patients in group 3 who had one or more affected sibs and are presumed to fall into a high-risk category designated "previsionally private syndrome." The genetic causes of familial occurrence in group 4 may represent segregation of a mendelian (most likely autosomal recessive) gene or of a submicroscopic chromosome rearrangement; in the former case, unaffected sibs have a negligibly small risk of having similarly affected children, but in the latter case that risk is as high as that of their parents.

The patients in group 3, by definition, all have physical examination syndromes, those in groups 1 and 4 have causal genesis syndromes, but many in group 2 have formal genesis syndromes, ie represent two or more idiopathic, sporadic cases with an apparently identical MCA/MR syndrome. Strictly speaking, the Rubinstein-Taybi syndrome is not a causally defined but only a formal genesis syndrome.

In this paper we report two sporadic patients with the same, previously apparently undescribed MCA/MR syndrome, initially considered a formal genesis syndrome since lymphocyte chromosomes were always apparently normal, but presently determined to be a causal genesis syndrome of group 1, since both were found to have the identical chromosome abnormality in their fibroblasts.

*Studies of Malformation Syndromes of Man XLIIC

Birth Defects: Original Article Series, Volume XIII, Number 3B, pages 103–110
© 1977 The National Foundation

CLINICAL REPORTS

We are reporting on a 37-year-old man and a 19-year-old woman (Figs. 1 and 2) who were long-time patients of P.D. Pallister at the Boulder River School and Hospital, Boulder, Montana, where they were studied annually for some 10 years by a number of medical geneticists who agreed in the main that these patients probably had an MCA/MR syndrome and that they both, with minor variations, had the identical syndrome. However, because of the paucity of major anomalies and the repeated apparent normality of the lymphocyte chromosomes it was also considered possible that the patients had a metabolic dysplasia syndrome and thus skin biopsies were taken from both that led to the discovery, by the Wisconsin State Laboratory of Hygiene (L. F. Meisner) of an extra chromosome in these fibroblasts.

Both patients are profoundly mentally retarded and bedridden, lack speech and all self-help skills, are peculiarly lethargic or somnolent, and have intermittent grand mal convulsions. Both have an essentially unremarkable family history. The woman was born after an unremarkable 45 week gestation when her mother and father were 32 and 44 years old, respectively. She weighed 4,100 gm at birth. The man was born normally, at term, with a birthweight of

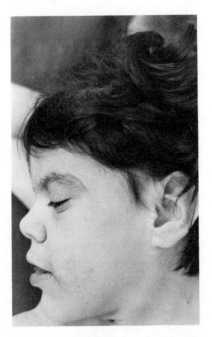 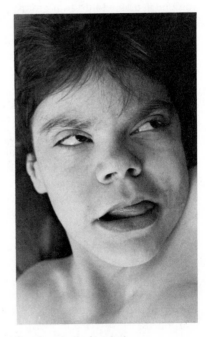

Fig. 1. *Patient 1* at 19 years; see text for phenotypic description.

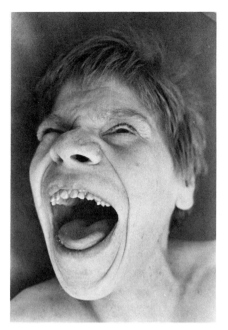

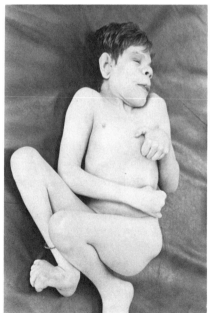
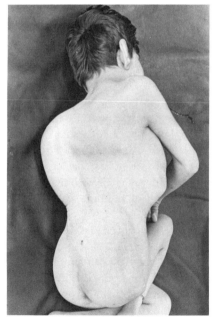

Fig. 2. *Patient 2* at 37 years; see text for phenotypic description. Note large, wedge-shaped patch of pigment on right lateral hip area.

3,211 gm and length of 53.5 cm. The neonatal periods were unremarkable, but both were noted to be severely to profoundly retarded in early childhood.

The man has a normal head circumference, but the girl is microcephalic; both are only 144 cm tall. The man has undetectable testes but otherwise normal genitalia. His secondary sexual characteristics are immature; he has some pubic hair. The girl has normally developed female secondary characteristics. At 14 years she suffered a traumatic vaginal perforation; during the operation an infantile uterus had to be removed; the ovaries appeared normal and a biopsy showed numerous immature oocytes.

Both patients have a "coarse" facial appearance that resembles that of patients on long-term diphenylhydantoin treatment; neither patient is or has been treated with this drug for a long time. Both have apparent telecanthus/hypertelorism, a broad, large nose with many small comedones at its tip, hirsute forehead, synophrys, broad eyebrows with ectopic eyelash or eyebrow hairs on the upper lids, mongoloid slanting of the palpebral fissures, hypoplasia of helix and prominence of lower antihelix and other minor anomalies of the auricles, macrostomia, and macroglossia (which may in part represent the effect of long-term rumination and chewing on hands); both lack several teeth and have widely spaced teeth; but the man also has gemination of the right lower lateral incisor. The palates are normal. The corneas are borderline small and have a slightly elliptical shape, with the blunt end pointing nasally; both have cataracts in both eyes, detectable only with ophthalmoscope and after dilation of the pupils in the girl, but grossly evident in the man, who has a dense cataract, miosis, increased depth of anterior chamber, and keratoconus in the right eye.

Both have widespread pigmentary dysplasia of the skin, clinically evident in the girl but barely noticeable in the man; this becomes very obvious under ultraviolet light in a dark room when the entire body becomes marbled and streaked in an incontinentia pigmenti-like manner. The man has many, the girl a few, pigmented moles and nevi.

Both have a severe dorsal kyphoscoliosis with compensatory lumbar curve, eversion of sacrum and coccyx with shallow gluteal cleft and sacral dimple, thoracic protuberance with retroversion of a cleft xiphisternum, subluxation of the left hip with multiple, passive flexion contractures of limbs and deformities of feet.

The young woman has 3 extra nipples above each breast and asymmetric breast size. She has a simian crease on the left palm, a bilateral t'' triradius, bilateral 3rd and right 4th interdigital distal loops, 6 ulnar loops, 3 arches and one whorl on the fingertips. He has bilateral t and t'' triradii with hypothenar ulnar loop, vestigial 3rd interdigital distal loops, and 7 whorls, 2 ulnar loops, and an arch on the fingertips.

Their muscles are atrophic and deep tendon reflexes are symmetrically hypoactive; however, in both, the muscles are more severely contracted on the left.

In both patients heart, lungs, and intravenous pyelograms were normal.

Skeletal roentgenograms confirmed clinical impressions and in the girl showed foreshortened vertebral bodies, decreased transverse diameter of pelvis with a narrow pelvic inlet and relative lack of iliac flare, subluxated and flattened left femoral head, bilateral valgus position of the femoral necks and decreased width of the shafts of the tubular bones. The metaphyses of the metacarpals and of the proximal humeri are slightly undermodeled. Her bone age is retarded and corresponds to 13.5 years. The man had similar findings with a thick calvarium and small neurocranium, wide paranasal sinuses, and marked shortness of the 1st and mild shortness of the 4th metacarpals.

Both have a highly abnormal EEG with generalized dysrhythmia.

Multiple lymphocyte cytogenetic studies performed on both over a 10-year span at Boulder consistently showed apparently normal chromosomes. Initial karyotypes from fibroblasts showed an extra "F-like" chromosome in 9 of 18 in the male patient and in 9 of 30 cells in the female patient. Studies of many additional cells with different banding techniques confirmed mosaicism with the aneuploid cell line in about half of her fibroblasts and a third of his. The extra chromosome was initially thought to be a chromosome 20 [2], but further banding studies have made it clear that the extra chromosome is not an F but derived from a 12. G, R and BSG [9] banding patterns are difficult to interpret. Two hypotheses have been considered: 1) The extra chromosome is an isochromosome of the short arm of 12 (Francke), or 2) it is a 12 with a partial deletion of the long arm (del [12] [pter→q13] Elejalde) (Fig. 3). Further studies are in progress in La Jolla and Madison to settle this question.

DISCUSSION

These two patients have a virtually identical, previously undefined and presumably rare MCA/deformity/MR syndrome; both have a previously undescribed chromosome abnormality; hence we conclude that the chromosome abnormality is the cause of the patients' condition. Prolonged postnatal survival presumably reflects mosaicism with normal cells.

The clinical data, and the fact that the mosaicism was present in all subcultures established in duplicate from three different biopsies obtained at different times, show convincingly 1) that the mosaicism did not arise in vitro but was present in the patients, that is, represents developmental mixoploidy, and 2) that the aneuploid cell line was probably responsible for the patients' abnormalities [3, 4]. The remarkable mosaicism found in these two cases is not unprecedented, but it prevented the identification of the correct cause of our patients' condition for many years until routine cytogenetic study of the fibroblast lines established from these patients (and intended for storage for future study) detected the aneuploid cell line.

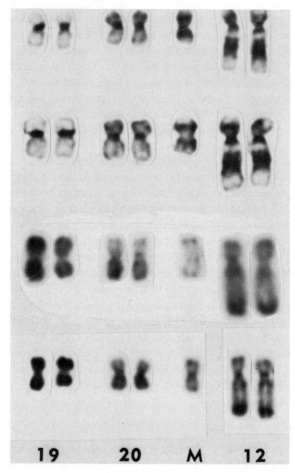

Fig. 3. Partial karyotypes of aneuploid cells from the female patient. Chromosomes in the first two rows were prepared with trypsin-Giemsa (G) banding (Francke) and in the bottom two rows with BSG banding (Elejalde). The supernumerary small metacentric chromosome is marked "M."

The cytogenetic interpretation of additional chromosome 12 material in the aneuploid cell line is supported by the three published studies on trisomy 12p due to translocation [5–7]. Clinical similarities include absence of intrauterine growth retardation, "flat facies," bilateral epicanthic folds, apparent hypertelorism, "broad and irregular implantation of the eyebrows (covering part of the upper eyelid)," large philtrum, broad and thick lower lip, prominence of antihelix, sacral dimple, hypotonia, severe MR and abnormal EEG (with seizures in the patient of Uchida and Lin [5]). The polymastia observed by Armendares et al [7] was interpreted by them as a coincidental autosomal dominant trait segregating in the father's family; however, from the evidence of our female patient it is more likely a component manifestation of duplications involving the short arm of 12. Again, no major congenital anomalies were observed in any of the patients in three previously reported families; cataracts were not mentioned, and the only skin anomaly reported was a hyperkeratosis in the patient of Armendares et al. However, the pigmentary disturbance can be subtle and may have been overlooked. The patient of Rethoré et al [6] also had a postaxial hexadactyly of the left foot and severe bilateral hydronephrosis, not seen in our patients.

When the cause of the syndrome in our two patients became evident, we restudied with Dr. Elisabeth G. Kaveggia at Central Wisconsin Colony in Madison a 36-year-old, severely retarded male with some minor anomalies and incontinentia pigmenti-like pigmentary dysplasia of the skin; he had been classified in the "primary seizure" group because of severe epilepsy, the minor nature of his other anomalies, and the fact that his lymphocyte chromosomes were apparently normal. Reexamination of this patient suggested strongly that he had the same syndrome that was present in the two Boulder patients. Studies of his fibroblasts confirmed that he had the same chromsome constitution with the extra small metacentric chromosome being present in 70% of metaphases. The University of Wisconsin dermatologists were impressed by similarities of this patient's skin pigmentary lesion to the entity designated "incontinentia pigmenti achromians" or "hypomelanosis of Ito" [8]. A review of the literature on this topic by Jelinek et al [8] suggests that the entity is heterogeneous (an autosomal dominant form seems to exist) and may be associated with "saddle nose," hypertelorism, mental retardation, EEG abnormality, hypotonia, "congenital luxation of the coccyx," permanent flexion deformity, facial hypertrichosis, thick lips, congenital hydronephrosis (see case of Rethoré et al [6]). We think that fibroblast chromosome studies of retarded, sporadic cases of Ito's hypomelanosis may show some of them to have the same chromosome constitution which was observed in our patients.

Thus we have shown 1) that there exists a characteristic malformation/deformity/mental retardation-seizure syndrome that is caused by the presence of a cell line with 47,+i (12p) or 47, del(12) (pter→q13) chromosome abnormality; and 2) that in spite of the somewhat subjective aspects of the delineation, this syndrome is so characteristic that it can be searched for successfully in at-risk populations. Our previous interpretation of F-trisomy due to postfertilization nondisjunction has to be revised on the basis of the new chromosome findings. The resolution of the cytologic nature of the extra chromosome may help in thinking about the most likely mechanism and time of its origin. During development after fertilization, apparent selection occurs against the aneuploid cell line in lymphocyte precursors. Fibroblasts of malformation/mental retardation patients formerly found to have apparently normal lymphocyte chromosomes may finally yield the cause of their condition, ie the presence of an aneuploid cell line.

ACKNOWLEDGMENTS

This work was supported, in part, by DHEW/PHS grants GM20130 and GM 21110 (to U.F.) from the National Institute of General Medical Sciences. Contributed, in part, as Paper No. 2043 from the University of Wisconsin Genetics Laboratory.

REFERENCES

1. Opitz JM: Diagnostic/genetic studies in severe mental retardation. In Lubs HA, de la Cruz F (eds): "Genetic Counseling." New York: Raven Press, 1977, pp 417–443.
2. Pallister PD, Herrmann J, Meisner LF, Inhorn SL, Opitz JM: Trisomy 20 syndrome in man. [Studies of malformation syndromes of man 43A.] Lancet 1:431, 1976.
3. Benn PA, Harnden DG: Trisomy 20 syndrome in man. Lancet 1:541, 1976.
4. Meisner LF, Pallister PD, Inhorn SL, Herrmann J, Opitz JM: Developmental mixoploidy and trisomy 20 syndrome. [Studies of malformation syndromes of man 43B.] Lancet 1:920, 1976.
5. Uchida IA, Lin CC: Identification of partial 12 trisomy by quinacrine fluorescence. J Pediatr 82:269–272, 1973.
6. Rethoré M-O, Kaplan J-C, Junien C, Cruveiller J, Dutrillaux B, Aurias A, Carpentier S, Lafourcade J, Lejeune J: Augmentation de l'activité de la LDH-B chez un garçon trisomique 12p par malségrégation d'une translocation maternèlle t(12;14) (q12;p11). Ann Génét 18:81–87, 1975.
7. Armendares S, Salamanca F, Nava S, Ramirez S, Cantu J-M: The 12p trisomy syndrome. Ann Génét 18:89–94, 1975.
8. Jelinek JE, Bart RS, Schiff GM: Hypomelanosis of Ito ("Incontinentia pigmenti achromians"). Report of three cases and review of the literature. Arch Dermatol 107:596–601, 1973.
9. Kanda M: Banding pattern observed in human chromosomes by the modified BSG technique. Hum Genet 31:283–292, 1976.

A Syndrome of Craniofacial, Digital, and Genital Anomalies

Mary Jo Harrod, PhD, Doman K. Keele, MD, and Jorge Howard, Sr, MD

An unusual complex of craniofacial, digital, and genital anomalies has been observed in two brothers and may represent a previously undescribed syndrome.

Diagnostic consultation and genetic counseling were requested by the parents of a 5-year-old, mentally retarded boy (*Case 1*) with multiple congenital anomalies during the mother's second pregnancy.

Case 1

A male child was born to a gravida 1 para 0 28-year-old mother after an uncomplicated pregnancy, labor, and delivery. At birth his weight was 2,650 gm, length was 53 cm, and head circumference was 33 cm. Multiple congenital anomalies were noted, including unusual facies, highly arched palate, large protruding ears, arachnodactyly, a small penis with penile hypospadias, and bilateral cryptorchidism. He was hospitalized at 4 weeks of age for failure to thrive and was found to have bilateral vocal cord paralysis with inspiratory stridor. Diagnostic laboratory studies included a normal male karyotype and normal blood and urine amino acids. Chest and skull roentgenograms were within normal limits, as was an upper GI series; he had an anomalous right subclavian artery. An IVP revealed minimal blunting of the calyces in the midportion of the right kidney and slight widening of the upper portion of the right ureter.

Subsequent growth was within normal limits except for weight, which continued at the 3rd percentile, due in part to feeding problems. His motor and intellectual development were markedly delayed. He sat without support at 12 months, crawled at 34 months, and walked at 38 months. At 20 months his vocabulary consisted of two words, and speech development lagged behind his other skills.

When seen for evaluation in 1974, at 5 years 10 months, he was an extremely thin (15.2 kg) retarded child with normal height (115 cm) and head circumference (50 cm). His skull was dolichocephalic and his facial appearance unusual (Fig. 1) with a long thin face, small pointed chin, apparent hypotelorism, pointed nose, and small mouth with malocclusion. His ears were large and anteverted. His palate was highly arched and his speech was nasal. Exotropia had been surgically corrected. His chest had a pigeon-breast deformity. His limbs were extremely thin. Striking arachnodactyly of all digits was present and cutaneous syndactyly was present between toes 2 and 3. A small penis with unrepaired hypospadias

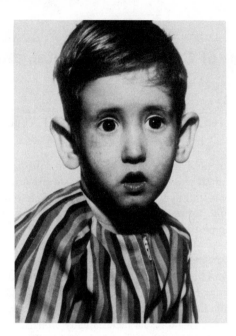

Fig. 1. *Case 1*. Age 5 years, 10 months.

was noted, as well as bilateral undescended testes. He had an IQ of 42 on the Stanford Binet scale, with his poorest functioning in vocabulary and verbal fluency. An audiometric examination was normal. A repeat lymphocyte karyotype with Giemsa banding was normal.

No diagnosis was possible; the parents were told that the pattern of anomalies did not suggest a recognizable syndrome and that the recurrence risk in such cases was usually low, but could be as high as 25% if an unrecognized single gene disorder was responsible. A second pregnancy resulted in the birth of a male infant with remarkably similar physical appearance and anomalies (*Case 2*).

Case 2

This boy was born after a normal term pregnancy and a labor and delivery complicated by a breech presentation. When hospitalized at 3 weeks of age for failure to thrive, he weighed 2,180 gm, was 49 cm long, and had a head circumference of 34 cm, all below the 3rd percentile. His facial appearance was remarkably similar to that of his brother (Figs. 2A and B) and similar anomalies of the limbs and genitalia were present.

All laboratory studies were reported as within normal limits, including a

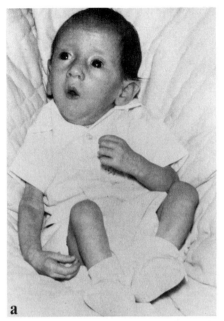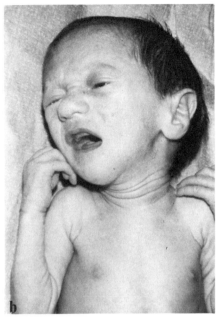

Fig. 2. a) *Case 1.* b) *Case 2.*

karyotype with Giemsa banding. Roentgenograms of the skull and chest were normal. An IVP showed vesicoureteral reflux on the left side and mild dilatation of the right kidney. A voiding cystourethrogram was normal.

The infant required gavage feeding. An upper GI series revealed hypertrophic pyloric stenosis. An aberrant right subclavian artery and malrotation of the small bowel were also noted.

The child died at 2 months of age before surgery could be carried out. Autopsy showed the abnormal facies, genital, and digital anomalies, but no anatomic cause of death; all organ systems were normal in appearance except for the pyloric stenosis, aberrant right subclavian artery, and multiple microcysts of the renal cortex.

DISCUSSION

The remarkable physical resemblance and similarity of clinical findings in these two brothers suggest a distinct dysmorphic syndrome, including craniofacial, digital, and genital anomalies. *Case 2* did not survive infancy. *Case 1* is retarded and has limited verbal ability. His speech problems are felt to be func-

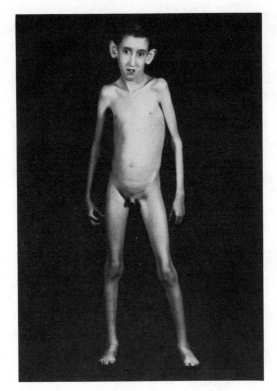

Fig. 3. *Case 1.*

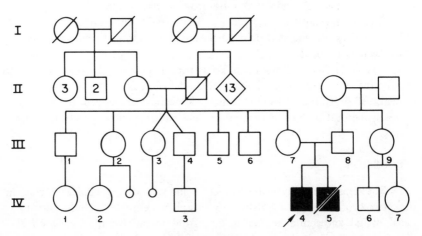

Fig. 4. Pedigree.

tional as well as anatomic. His physical appearance has become even more unusual with increasing age (Fig. 3). An initial diagnosis of the Smith-Lemli-Opitz syndrome [1] was considered, but the facial appearance of our patients does not resemble that described in patients with that disorder, and growth retardation and microcephaly are not present in our surviving patient.

The occurrence of this unusual combination of anomalies in two brothers is consistent with either autosomal recessive or X-linked recessive inheritance. There is no family history of similar anomalies and consanguinity is denied. Both of the mother's sisters have had unexplained miscarriages; her four brothers are alive and well (Fig. 4). The recognition of similar findings in other patients may lead to the delineation of the genetic nature of the syndrome and the provision of more satisfactory genetic counseling in such cases.

REFERENCES

1. Smith DW, Lemli L, Opitz JM: A newly recognized syndrome of multiple congenital anomalies. J Pediatr 64:210-217, 1964.

New Syndrome of Chronic Mucocutaneous Candidiasis*

Gary A. Okamoto, MD, Judith G. Hall, MD, Hans Ochs, MD,
Charles Jackson, MD, Keith Rodaway, MD, and John Chandler, MD

In this article we introduce a family which, we believe, represents a new type of chronic mucocutaneous candidiasis with dominant inheritance. It is characterized by an early onset, mild mucocutaneous candidiasis, increased susceptibility to bacterial infection, hyperkeratosis follicularis, alopecia universalis, keratoconjunctivitis, diarrhea in infancy, T and B-cell abnormalities, and possible hypoadrenalism. The affected family members whom we have studied are a mother and her two daughters. Their maternal grandfather was possibly affected.

CASE REPORTS

Case 1

A 28-year-old Caucasian gravida 4, para 2, abortus 2 woman was the 2,580 gm term product of an uncomplicated pregnancy and delivery. Although her growth was normal, she developed bilateral keratoconjunctivitis with hazy and markedly vascularized corneas at 5 yr; this was preceded by photophobic symptoms for 2 yr (Fig. 1). When a teenager, she became legally blind and developed cataracts. As an infant, she had blonde, wiry, dry, long hair that fell out gradually and completely by age 15 necessitating use of a wig as early as 6 yr of age. Menarche and breast development were normal, but she failed to grow axillary and pubic hair. She is of normal intelligence and graduated from high school despite being teased and ostracized.

Chronic mucocutaneous candidiasis began at about age 5 as did vulvitis and inflammation at the corners of the mouth. On several occasions, severe monilial vulvovaginitis was complicated by bacterial infection leading to hospitalization. Chronic monilial nail infection began in her late teens. After puberty, she

*This research was supported by the Gene Center grant GM15253 from the U.S. Public Health Service.

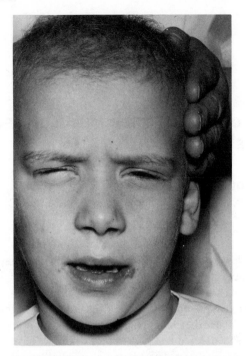

Fig. 1. Squinting and photophobia from interstitial keratitis and lesions at the corners of the mouth in mother at 6.5 years of age.

experienced bacterial cellulitis, cutaneous abscesses, recurrent urinary tract infection, pneumonia, paronychia and mastitis (Fig. 2). These bacterial infections have responded well to conventional antibiotic therapy.

On physical examination she appeared as an alert, stocky, bald, and blind woman (Fig. 3). Minimal conjunctival injection, marked corneal haziness and vascularization, and surgical aphakia were present. The corners of her mouth were slightly inflamed and scaly. Her vulvar area was injected and moderately lichenified. Fingernails were thickened, splitting, and yellowish. Skin was dry, rough, and hairless. Examination of the thyroid gland, chest, abdomen, and lymph nodes were within normal limits.

Significant family history revealed that her father's skin had been rough, dry, and unusually tanned, even during winter (Fig. 5). His hair was wiry and normally distributed. He had progressive blindness during his 20s but had no history of recurrent infection. He died unexpectedly at 36 yr of age while recovering from bacterial pneumonia. On autopsy, his adrenal glands were of average

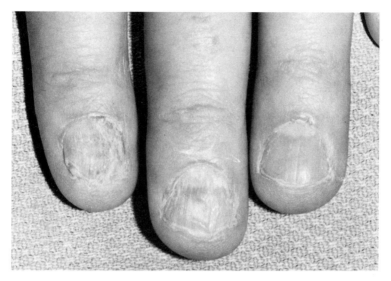

Fig. 2. Nail infection of mother.

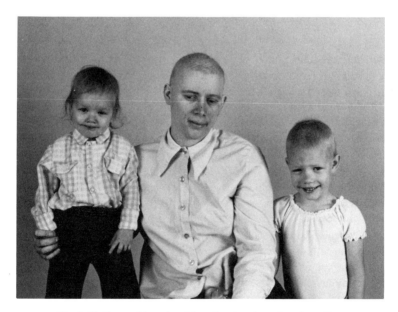

Fig. 3. Mother and two daughters showing alopecia universalis.

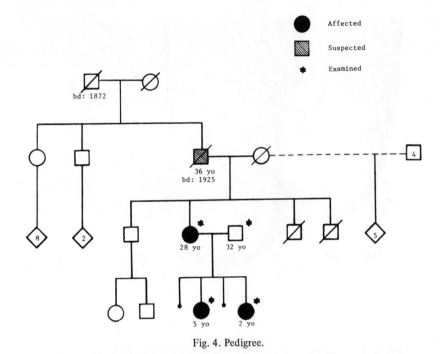

Fig. 4. Pedigree.

size with a borderline low normal cortical thickness of 2 mm. His own father was 52 yr old and his mother was in her mid 40s when he was born. Apparently, there are no other affected individuals.

The husband of *Case 1* is a 32-yr-old blind, obese Caucasian man with grand mal seizures, the victim of a recent myocardial infarction. His blindness was due to optic neuritis in childhood.

Case 2

The 5-yr-old daughter of *Case 1* was a 2,800 gm term infant delivered by cesarean section due to severe soft tissue and cervical dystocia. Development of progressive alopecia, photophobia, and bilateral keratoconjuncti-vitis with vascularization paralleled her mother's course. In late infancy, she experienced a month of unexplained watery diarrhea that remitted spontaneously. Except for inflammation at the corners of the mouth, she has not had nail or vulvar infection.

On physical examination, her length, weight, and head circumference were within normal limits. In bright light, she squinted and tilted her head down. On slit-lamp examination, keratoconjunctivitis with vascularization was present but there were no cataracts. Her skin was dry, rough, and hairless. Scalp hair was sparse, short, wiry and dry (Fig. 3). The rest of physical examination was normal.

Case 3

The 24-month-old daughter of *Case 1* was a 2,600 gm term product of an uncomplicated pregnancy and repeat cesarean section. During early infancy, dry rough skin was noted (Fig. 5). At 18 months she showed signs of keratoconjunctivitis with mild vascularization on slit-lamp biomicroscopy, and some thinning of her scalp hair. She was hospitalized twice for persistent watery diarrhea and severe Candida diaper dermatitis. Extensive evaluation of her intestinal tract failed to explain the diarrhea. Over the past 15 months, she has had several 4–6-week episodes of diarrhea that show inconsistent improvement with clear liquids or soy-bean formula.

On physical examination (Fig. 3), she had a normal length, weight, and head circumference. Skin texture, hair, and corneas were as described above. She had nasal discharge, decreased mobility of the tympanic membranes, and mild ammoniacal dermatitis. Language development was questionably delayed.

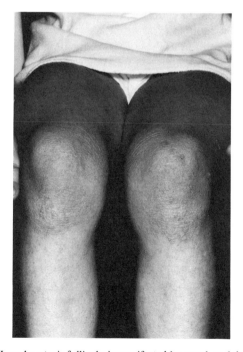

Fig. 5. Hyperkeratosis follicularis manifested by rough and dry skin.

METHODS AND RESULTS

Our evaluation focused on the immunologic, cutaneous, and endocrine aspects of the syndrome. Tests for T-cell function were abnormal. Although the mother and older daughter had positive cutaneous tests for delayed hypersensitivity to Candida, the younger daughter had a negative test in the face of culture-proven Candida dermatitis. This may represent true cutaneous anergy. In vitro lymphocyte transformation was depressed to nonspecific mitogens (phytohemagglutinin, Concanavalin A, and pokeweed) and allogene cells in mixed leukocyte cultures. Lymphocyte transformation to specific Candida antigen was very depressed. Absolute lymphocyte count and sheep erythrocyte rosette tests were normal.

B-cell function demonstrated subtle abnormalities. Serum Candida agglutinins were present at 1:4 to 1:32 titers, not extraordinarily elevated as often seen in chronic mucocutaneous candidiasis [1,2]. Candida antibodies in the saliva were absent in this family. Usually, patients with chronic candidiasis have detectable levels of antibodies in the saliva [1]. EAC-rosette formation was decreased. Phage ØX 174 immunization provoked low normal to low antibody responses after primary and secondary injections. Serum immunoglobulins (IgA, IgM, IgG, and IgE), isohemagglutinins, Coombs (direct and indirect) and absolute neutrophil count were normal.

Cumulatively, cultures of the corners of the mouth, nails, perineum, and vulvovaginal area have been positive for Candida species.

Results of other tests that were normal are as follows: hemoglobin, total white blood cell count, complement factors, nitroblue tetrazolium dye test, leukocyte myeloperoxidase, urinalysis, and chest x rays.

Because of the association between autoimmune endocrinopathy and chronic mucocutaneous candidiasis and the grandfather's ominous history, it seemed appropriate to perform an endocrine evaluation on the family [3,4]. The 24-hr urinary 17-hydroxysteroids were normal in the mother but slightly below normal in her older daughter. The 24-hr urinary 17-ketosteroids were normal. A metyrapone oral challenge produced only a slight rise in serum 11-deoxycortisol. Rather than attribute the subnormal response to a selective ACTH deficiency, we postulated that the metyrapone inhibition was ineffective. Therefore, to rule out adrenal insufficiency, a 4-hr ACTH infusion was performed and provoked a normal rise in the mother but a slightly less than the expected rise of serum cortisol in the older daughter [5]. Results of thyroid function tests, glucose tolerance tests, calcium, phosphorus, alkaline phosphatase, electrolytes, and blood urea nitrogen were normal.

Results of tests for seven different autoantibodies (including those against adrenal, parietal, and thyroid tissue) were negative in the sera.

We also suspected that the alopecia and hyperkeratosis follicularis were due to an autoimmune process partly because hair loss has been progressive and has occurred over noninfected areas of the skin. However, light microscopy and direct immunofluorescence (IgA, IgM, IgG, and complement) did not reveal lymphocyte or immunoglobulin aggregation in multiple skin biopsies. Hair shafts had normal morphology.

DISCUSSION

This family seems to be different from the usually reported syndromes involving chronic mucocutaneous candidiasis [6]. The features which make this family unique are dominant inheritance, alopecia universalis, progressive keratoconjunctivitis with corneal vascularization, and B-cell abnormalities.

GENETICS

The pedigree suggests autosomal dominant inheritance although X-linked dominant inheritance cannot be excluded (Fig. 4). The paternal great-grandfather was 52 years old when he had his son, suggesting possible new dominant mutation associated with advanced paternal age. By history, the maternal grandfather probably had a mild variant of the condition which he passed on to his daughter. Her two daughters obviously have the disorder. Previously reported patients with chronic mucocutaneous candidiasis have been sporadic cases or familial cases affecting only sibs, suggesting autosomal recessive inheritance.

NATURAL HISTORY

In this family, during infancy and early childhood, moniliasis occurred infrequently in the perineal region but once established, it was resistant to routine treatment. In later childhood, chronic vulvovaginitis, nail infection, and mouth lesions were a problem (Figs. 1 and 2). Interestingly, after puberty, the mother has apparently had increased susceptibility to bacterial infection. All three individuals have handled viral infections well, and immunizations have been given without complications.

The earliest identifiable feature of the syndrome was the rough, dry skin (Fig. 5) noted shortly after birth. Her hair was dry, wiry, and grew initially only to fall out gradually and completely by puberty (Fig. 3); she has never grown axillary or pubic hair.

Bilateral keratoconjunctivitis presented initially as photophobia at 2 or 3 years of age and progressed despite topical corticosteroid therapy (Fig. 1). Legal blindness and cataract formation ensued in the mother in her teens.

Unexplained, watery diarrhea was present in infancy in the two daughters and has been outgrown in the older one.

Judging from the known association between chronic candidiasis and hypo-adrenalism [3], the grandfather's medical history, and the slightly abnormal endocrine tests, we suspect that an insidious development of hypoadrenalism may be part of this syndrome.

While affected individuals were small for gestational age, postnatal growth as well as mental development have been normal.

HYPOTHESES

A unifying theory has not yet been proposed to explain the wide variability and heterogeneity of syndromes involving chronic mucocutaneous candidiasis. Nevertheless, a few observations apparent from the literature [1,3,4] and probably relevant to our family should be stated. First, Candida usually limits its infection to the skin and does not invade internal organs. This family lacked evidence of systemic Candida involvement. Second, chronic candidiasis is often associated with atrophic endocrinopathies with or without autoantibodies and usually precedes the development of glandular insufficiency by months or even years. In this family, despite the absence of detectable autoantibodies, there is laboratory evidence to suggest the early development of adrenal deterioration. Third, autoantibodies should be regarded as markers of tissue degeneration but, as in this family, the absent antibodies do not necessarily mean the absence of disease.

Although we lack the data to incriminate autoimmunity [7], it appears clinically that the intestinal tract, skin, hair follicles, and corneas might undergo such a process.

The T-cell defects are consistent with reports in the literature [1, 8] and probably reflect a peculiar host susceptibility to fungal infections. The role of B-cell function is not clearly understood in this family. The absent salivary antibodies against Candida may mean poor local defenses against the organism. The mild abnormalities in EAC-rosette formation and antibody response to $\emptyset$X 174 immunization are likewise difficult to interpret.

IMPLICATIONS

Because of the progressive nature of this condition, particularly loss of vision associated with keratoconjunctivitis, immunotherapy is presently being considered, such as a trial of transfer factor or levamisole [9–11]. Furthermore, the suspicious history and known association between endocrinopathies and chronic candidiasis warrant periodic surveillance of their endocrine functions.

ACKNOWLEDGMENTS

The authors gratefully acknowledge the technical assistance of Ellen Powers and Kathleen Wilson.

REFERENCES

1. Kirkpatrick CH, Rich RR, Bennett JE: Chronic mucocutaneous candidiasis: Model-building in cellular immunity. Ann Intern Med 74:955-978, 1971.
2. Chilgren RA, Meuwissen HJ, Quie PG, Hong R: Chronic mucocutaneous candidiasis, deficiency of delayed hypersensitivity, and selective local antibody defect. Lancet 2: 688-692, 1967.
3. Blizzard RM, Gibbs JH: Candidiasis: Studies pertaining to its association with endocrinopathies and pernicious anemia. Pediatrics 42:231-237, 1968.
4. Wuepper KD, Fudenberg HH: Moniliasis, autoimmune polyendocrinopathy, and immunologic family study. Clin Exp Immunol 2:71-82, 1967.
5. Melby JC: Assessment of adrenocortical function. N Engl J Med 285:735-739, 1971.
6. Higgs JM, Wells RS: Chronic mucocutaneous candidiasis: Associated abnormalities of iron metabolism. Br J Dermatol (Suppl)8:88-102, 1972.
7. Stiller CR, Russell AS, Dossetor JB: Autoimmunity: Present concepts. Ann Intern Med 82:405-410, 1975.
8. Ammann AJ, Hong R: Cellular immunodeficiency disorders. In Stiehm ER, Fulginiti VA (eds): "Immunologic Disorders in Infants and Children." Philadelphia: W.B. Saunders, 1973, Chap 15, pp 249-254.
9. Van Scoy RE, Hill HR, Ritts RE, Quie PG: Familial neutrophil chemotaxis defect, recurrent bacterial infections, mucocutaneous candidiasis, and hyperimmunoglobulinemia. Ann Intern Med 82:766-771, 1975.
10. Wong VG, Kirkpatrick CH: Immune reconstitution in keratoconjunctivitis and superficial candidiasis. Arch Ophthalmol 92:335-339, 1974.
11. Kirkpatrick CH, Smith TS: Chronic mucocutaneous candidiasis: Immunologic and antibiotic therapy. Ann Intern Med 80:310-320, 1974.

Two "New" Autosomal Recessive Mental Retardation Syndromes Observed Among the Amish

Andrew N. Gale, MB, ChB, MRCP, Yves Lacassie, MD,
John G. Rogers, MB, BS, DCH, FRACP, L. Stefan Levin, DDS, MSD,
and Victor A. McKusick, MD

The clinical [1], cytologic [2, 3], and dermatoglyphic [4, 5] features of the Down syndrome are well established. It is doubtful that the diagnosis is acceptable in the absence of trisomy 21 or partial trisomy 21. Familial cases of the Down syndrome may be due to translocation [6] of part of chromosome 21. It is likely that trisomy of the distal segment of the long arm of chromosome 21 alone produces the syndrome [7–9].

We report two Amish sibships each with a different autosomal recessive syndrome that has some features of the Down syndrome.

CASE REPORTS

Family I

The parents of this sibship had at least 12 common ancestral couples (Fig. 1) and a coefficient of consanguinity of 0.03. There were two affected sisters, and a normal 9-year-old brother. No other family members were known to be affected.

Case I.1. The mother of this 18-year-old white female was 23 and the father 25 at the time of her birth. Pregnancy was uneventful and she was delivered at term after breech presentation. Birthweight was 2,211 gm and length was 46 cm. A diagnosis of the Down syndrome was made by her local physician when she was 2 days old. Her development was severely retarded. She crawled at about 2.5 years and walked at 8 years. She has never acquired speech or understanding of the spoken word, nor is she toilet-trained. Since 2 years of age, she has had seizures for which she has been treated with diphenylhydantoin and phenobarbital. Spinal

Birth Defects: Original Article Series, Volume XIII, Number 3B, pages 127–138
© 1977 The National Foundation

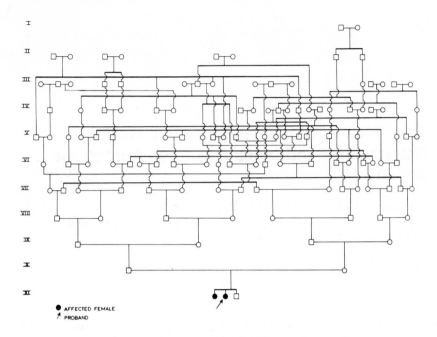

Fig. 1. Pedigree of *Family 1*.

fluid and electroencephalogram at 9 years showed no abnormalities. She has never menstruated. On psychometric testing at 12.5 years she had a perceptive language age of 32 weeks and an expressive language age of 20 weeks. Physical features at 7 years are shown in Figure 2.

At 18 years, on physical examination the proband, severely mentally retarded, aggressive, and uncooperative, was 142 cm tall, weighed 40 kg, and had a head circumference of 52 cm — all of these measurements were below the third percentile for age and sex (Fig. 3). Her occiput was flattened and her neck was thick. There was a mongoloid slant of the palpebral fissures, mild epicanthic folds but no Brushfield spots. She had horizontal nystagmus and high myopia. The tongue was large and fissured; it protruded from an open mouth and there was considerable drooling. The palate was narrow. The ears were normal in position and configuration. The sternum was short and there was a mild Harrison sulcus. There was a soft, short, systolic murmur in the second left intercostal space. The hands were small and the fingers were fat proximally and tapered distally (Fig. 4a). There was bilateral clinodactyly but no simian line. The toes were short with a wide space between the hallux and 2nd toe. Joints were moderately lax but the elbows and knees were not hyperextensible. There was a marked lumbar lordosis (Fig. 3), bilateral genu valgum, pes planus, and eversion of both feet. Muscle tone, deep tendon reflexes, and plantar responses were normal. External genitalia were normal and she

was at stage 3 of puberty [10]. No abdominal organs were palpable. Hearing
was normal. Urine contained no amino acids or mucopolysaccharides.

Case I. 2. This 19-year-old severely retarded female was the sister of *Case I.1.*
There was a three-day episode of bleeding in the first trimester of pregnancy.
Iron tablets were the only drugs taken during the pregnancy and delivery was
normal after spontaneous labor at 38 weeks. The baby weighed 2,155 gm at birth,
and she remained in the hospital for 3 weeks because of low birthweight. The
neonatal period was otherwise uncomplicated. Development was severely retarded. She walked at 3 years but has never acquired speech or toilet-training.
At 3 years she developed edema and proteinuria and a diagnosis of nephrotic
syndrome was made. Recurrent exacerbations have responded to steroids and
diuretics. Since 5.5 years she has had grand mal seizures for which she has been

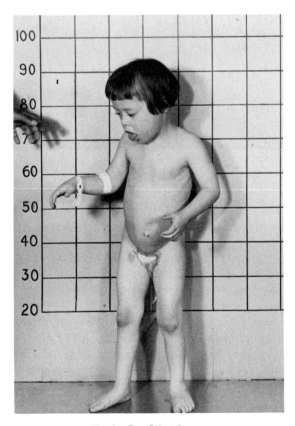

Fig. 2. *Case I.1* at 7 years.

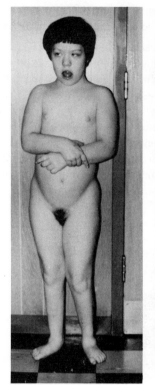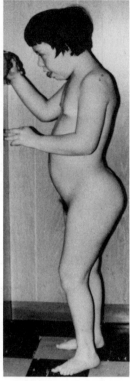

Fig. 3. *Case I.1* at 18 years.

treated with diphenylhydantoin and phenobarbital. At 8 years EEG was grossly abnormal with moderate- to high voltage multifocal spike discharges maximal in the right temporal region. Spinal fluid examination and motor and sensory nerve conduction velocities were normal. She has never menstruated. Psychometric testing at 4 years, 11 months had given a perceptive language age of 40 weeks and an expressive language age of 28 weeks.

On examination she was found to be a severely mentally retarded white female who resembled her sister in appearance and behavior. The physical features at 8 years are shown in Figure 5. At 19 years, she was 142 cm tall, weighed 38 kg, and her head circumference was 51 cm; all these measurements are below the 3rd percentile for her age and sex. There was a mongoloid slant of the palpebral fissures with epicanthic folds (Fig. 6), myopia, and horizontal nystagmus. She had marked gingival hypertrophy, presumably due to diphenylhydantoin therapy and poor dental hygiene. The palate was narrow and the tongue was fissured. There

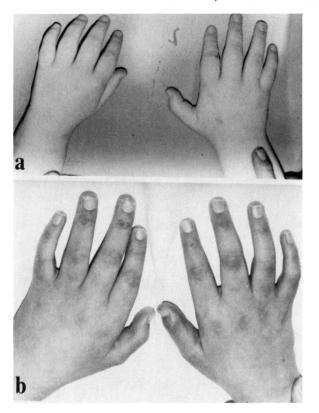

Fig. 4. a) Hands of *Case I.1;* b) hands of *Case I.2.* The tapering fingers are present in both but more marked in the former.

were no Brushfield spots and the ears were normal in position and configuration. The sternum was short and she had mild pectus excavatum. The joints were lax. Muscle tone was normal; reflexes were present and equal and plantar responses were flexor. The fingers were fat proximally and tapered distally (Fig. 4b). There was no simian line or clinodactyly. The external genitalia were normal, and she was in stage 4 of puberty [10]. The heart was normal and no abdominal organs were palpable.

Urine contained no amino acids or mucopolysaccharides. An intravenous pyelogram at 19 years was normal.

Peripheral blood lymphocytes from the proband, her sister, parents, and brother were cultured by standard methods. Karyotypes were examined using G- and Q-banding, and R-banding was done on the proband. No abnormalities of chromosome number or structure were found.

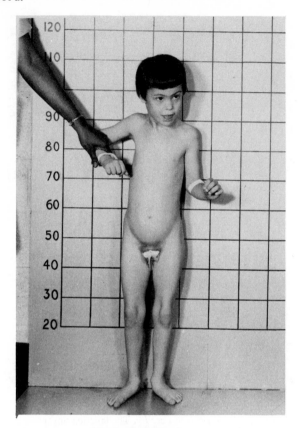

Fig. 5. *Case I.2* at 8 years.

Family II

The parents of these three affected sibs were Amish and had a coefficient of consanguinity of 0.04 (Fig. 7). No other close relatives were known to be affected. There were four normal sibs.

Case II.1. This was a 42-year-old, severely mentally retarded female (Fig. 8). She had recently developed diabetes mellitus, controlled with chlorpropamide. She had had a cholecystectomy at 18 years. She helped with chores around the home and spent much of her time sewing. She understood simple language but speech was limited to a few incoherent words. She menstruated regularly.

She was 143 cm tall, which is below the third percentile. She was obese and the facial features were coarse (Fig. 9a). There was an antimongoloid slant of the palpebral fissures, which were also narrow. There was keratoconus on the left and

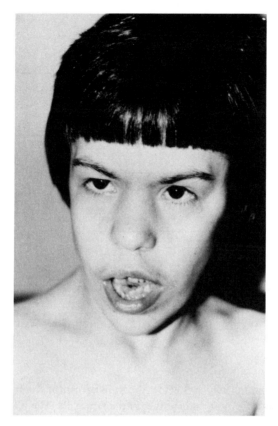

Fig. 6. *Case I.2* at 19 years.

an early cataract on the right. The nose was broad and the auricles were rotated posteriorly but were otherwise normal. The maxillary canines were absent. She had bilateral clinodactyly, a left transitional simian crease, hypothenar flexion creases bilaterally, and an adduction deformity of both thumbs. The toes were short with overlapping 5th toes bilaterally. The knees were hyperextensible. Muscle tone was normal, reflexes were brisk apart from the ankle jerks, which were depressed. Plantar responses were normal and the heart was normal.

Case II.2. The 36-year-old brother of *Case II.1* was also severely mentally retarded and resembled his sister (Fig. 9b). He too understood spoken words but did not speak coherently. He was prone to temper tantrums, each lasting only a few minutes, but he was not violent. He led a useful life, helping on the farm.

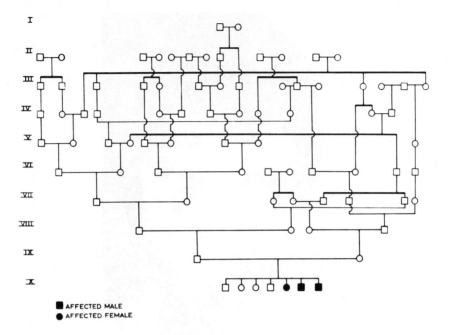

I

II

III

IV

V

VI

VII

VIII

IX

X

■ AFFECTED MALE
● AFFECTED FEMALE

Fig. 7. Pedigree of *Family 2*.

He was 147 cm tall, which is below the third percentile. He had a lipoma over the bridge of the nose and another in the left axilla. The facial features were coarse and he had an antimongoloid slant of the palpebral fissues and Brushfield spots. The ears were normal but the nose was broad. The maxillary left central incisor was tapered and had a vertical ridge of enamel on its labial surface. Two teeth were missing in the maxillary anterior region. The tooth in the position of the lower right 1st premolar had a star-shaped occlusal surface. He had clino-dactyly and hypothenar flexion creases bilaterally. The feet were short; there was wide separation of the 1st and 2nd toes, pes cavus, and an overlapping left 5th toe. He was not hypotonic and the deep tendon reflexes were all brisk with normal plantar responses. The heart was normal.

Case II.3. The youngest member of this sibship (Fig. 9c), aged 34 years, was less severely affected than the others, although his speech was severely limited.

He was 151 cm tall, which is just below the third percentile, and his facial features resembled those of his affected sibs, although they were not so coarse. He had an antimongoloid slant to the eyes, and frontal bossing. The ears were rotated posteriorly about 30° and the nose was broad. The teeth were normal. He had bilateral clinodactyly and a transverse hypothenar flexion crease on the right. The feet were short with pes cavus and an overriding 5th toe bilaterally.

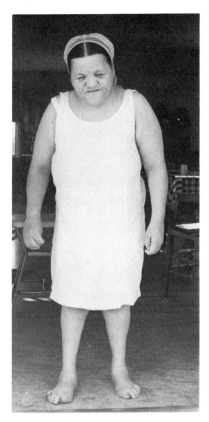

Fig. 8. *Case II.1* at 43 years.

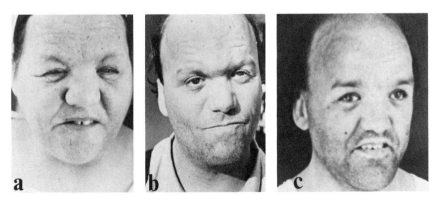

Fig. 9. Facial features of a) *Case II.1*, b) *Case II.2*, and c) *Case II.3*.

There was an umbilical hernia. The heart was normal as was the muscle tone, but the deep tendon reflexes were brisk. Plantar responses were normal.

Mucopolysaccharides and abnormal amino acids were absent from the urine in all three sibs. Giemsa-banded karyotypes of the three affected individuals and their phenotypically normal father were normal.

DERMATOGLYPHICS

The results of dermatoglyphic analysis are shown in Table 1. The Hopkins composite (log odd) score is derived from the data shown by the method described by Bolling et al [11]. In normal subjects the scores are negative; in the Down syndrome scores are positive. None of the scores we obtained were positive.

DISCUSSION

Both the sibships we have described are the products of consanguineous marriages in a highly inbred group. This fact and the involvement of more than one sib suggest that each of these syndromes is an autosomal recessive trait, and

Table 1. Dermatoglyphic Patterns in Families I and II.

	Family I				Family II					
	Case I.1		Case I.2		Case II.1		Case II.2		Case II.3	
	L	R	L	R	L	R	L	R	L	R
Hallucal	L^d	L^D	L^d	L^d	L^d	W	W^s	W	W	W
Great toe	L^f	L^f	L^t	L^t	L^f	L^f	L^f	L^f	L^f	L^f
Palmar interdigital I	–	–	–	–	–	–	–	–	–	–
Palmar interdigital II	–	–	–	–	–	–	–	–	–	–
Palmar interdigital III	–	L^d	L^d	L^d	L^d	–	–	–	–	L^d
Palmar interdigital IV	L^d	L^d	L^d	L^d	L^d	L^d	L^d	L^d	L^d	–
Palmar axial triradius	t'	t'	t'	t'	t	t	t	t	t''	t''
Hypothenar	–	–	–	–	–	–	–	–	L^u	W
Simian crease	–	–	–	–	–	–	–	–	–	–
5th finger flexion crease	2	2	2	2	2	2	2	2	2	2
Finger I	L^u	L^u	L^u	L^u	L^u	L^u	L^u	L^u	L^u	L^u
II	L^r	A	A	A	W	W	L^r	L^r	L^r	L^r
III	A	L^u	A	A	L^u	L^u	L^u	L^u	L^u	L^u
IV	L^u	L^u	L^u	L^u	L^u	W	L^u	L^u	L^u	L^u
V	L^u	L^u	L^u	L^u	L^u	L^u	L^u	L^u	L^u	L^u
Hopkins composite score	– 2.48		– 6.22		–7.99		– 8.52		– 1.57	

Definitions: – = absence of pattern; L^t = loop tibial; L^f = loop fibular; L^d = loop distal, ridge count < 20; L^D = loop distal, ridge count > 20; L^u = loop ulnar; L^r = loop radial; A = arch; W = whorl; W^s = whorl with seam; t = 0–15%; t' = 16–40%; t'' = 40%.

the finding of normal karyotypes is consistent with that hypothesis. Many autosomal recessive traits have been described in the Amish [12–16], and it is perhaps surprising, considering the high degree of consanguinity and the large average family size in this population [17], that no other similar cases have been found.

ACKNOWLEDGMENTS

This study was supported by NIH Training grant GM00795. Andrew N. Gale was in receipt of a Wellcome Research Travel grant.

We thank Dr. A. Reyes and the staff at Ebensberg State School and Hospital, Ebensberg, Pennsylvania, for their cooperation, Dr. D. S. Borgaonkar and his staff for assistance with karyotype and dermatoglyphic studies, Dr. G. H. Thomas for carrying out metabolic studies, Mr. David Bolling for assistance with the Amish genealogy, Mrs. B. J. Latrobe for drawing the pedigrees, and Mrs. A. Sahm and Miss S. Schofield for typing the manuscript.

REFERENCES

1. Penrose LS: Mongolism. Br Med Bull 17:184–189, 1961.
2. Lejeune J, Gautier M, Turpin R: Étude des chromosomes somatiques de neuf enfants mongoliens. CR Acad Sci [D] (Paris) 248:1721–1722, 1959.
3. Casperson T, Hultén M, Lindsten J, Zech L.: Distinction between extra G-like chromosomes by quinacrine mustard fluorescence analysis. Exp Cell Res 63:240–243, 1970.
4. Cummins H: Dermatoglyphic stigmata in mongoloid imbeciles. Anat Rec 73:407–415, 1939.
5. Turpin R, Lejeune J: Étude dermatoglyphique des paumes des mongoliens et de leurs parents et germains. Sém Hôp Paris 76:3955–3967, 1953.
6. Williams JD, Summitt RL, Martens PR, Kimbrell RA: Familial Down syndrome due to t(10;21) translocation: evidence that the Down phenotype is related to trisomy of a specific segment of chromosome 21. Am J Hum Genet 27:478–485, 1975.
7. Niebuhr R: Down syndrome: The possibility of a pathogenetic segment on chromosome no 21. Humangenetik 21:99–101, 1974.
8. Sinet PM, Couturier J, Dutrillaux B. Poissonnier M, Raoul O. Rethore MD, Allard D, Lejeune J, Jerome H: Trisomie 21 et superoxyde dismutase-1 (IPO-A). Tentative de localisation sur la sous bande 21q22.1. Exp Cell Res 97:47–55, 1976.
9. Poissonnier M, Saint-Paul B, Dutrillaux B, Chassagne M, Gruyer P, Blignieres-Strouk G de: Trisomie 21 partielle (21q21→21q22.2) Ann Genet (Paris) 19:69–73, 1976.
10. Tanner JM: "Growth and Adolescence." 2nd Ed. Oxford and Edinburgh: Blackwell Scientific Publications, 1962.
11. Bolling DR, Borgaonkar DS, Herr HM, Davis M: Evaluation of dermal patterns in Down's syndrome by predictive discrimination. II. Composite score based on the combination of left and right pattern areas. Clin Genet 2:163–169, 1971.
12. Jackson LE, Carey JH: Progressive muscular dystrophy: Autosomal recessive type. Pediatrics 28:77–84, 1961.
13. McKusick VA, Egeland JA, Eldridge R, Krusen DE: Dwarfism in the Amish. I. The Ellis van Creveld syndrome. Bull Johns Hopk Hosp 115:306–336, 1964.

14. McKusick VA, Eldridge R, Hostetler JA, Ruanguit U, Egeland JA: Dwarfism in the Amish. II. Cartilage-hair hypoplasia. Bull Johns Hopk Hosp 116:285–326, 1965.
15. Cross HE, McKusick VA: The Mast syndrome: A recessively inherited form of presenile dementia with motor disturbances. Arch Neurol 16:1–13, 1967.
16. Cross HE, McKusick VA: The Troyer syndrome. A recessive form of spastic paraplegia with distal muscle wasting. Arch Neurol 16:473–485, 1967.
17. Hostetler JA: "Amish Society." Baltimore: The Johns Hopkins Press, 1963.

A Distinct Skeletal Dysplasia in an Infant From Consanguineous Parents

José María Cantú, MD, Carlos Manzano, MD, Praddy Pagán, BSc,
Diana García-Cruz, MD, and Alejandro Hernández, MD

We studied an infant with a previously undescribed set of skeletal anomalies consisting mainly of short-limb dwarfism, craniofacial disproportion, and platyspondyly. Although the case is sporadic, the clinical characteristics and the parental consanguinity suggest that the syndrome could be an autosomal recessive trait.

CASE REPORT

The male infant (*IV-17* in Fig. 1), was the product of a third, full-term, uncomplicated pregnancy and normal delivery. Birthweight was 3.2 kg; the length was not recorded, but the parents were informed that the patient looked short. Psychomotor development has been within low normal limits; an IQ of 75 was determined at 5 yr.

At 3½ years his weight was 10.5 kg and height 72.5 cm ($<$ 3%) [1]. The cephalic, thoracic, and abdominal circumferences were 49, 47.5 and 49 cm, respectively. The U/L segment ratio was 1.58 (44.5/28), which is above the 97th percentile.

The skull was dolichocephalic with prominent forehead. There were bilateral epicanthal folds and entropion (which have caused chronic conjunctivitis and secondary leukoma), short nose with mildly depressed nasal bridge, and mild micrognathia. The ears were large and low-set but normally differentiated. The neck was short as was the trunk; there was a marked pectus carinatum and the sternum was short. The abdomen was protuberant and there was hepatomegaly (5.4 and 2.5 cm in conventional lines below the costal edges) and splenomegaly (1.5 cm below the left costal edge). The genitalia were normal; both testes were

Birth Defects: Original Article Series, Volume XIII, Number 3B, pages 139–147

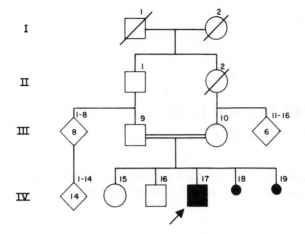

Fig. 1. Pedigree.

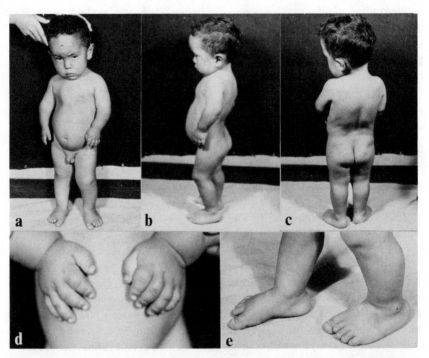

Fig. 2. The propositus at 3½ years of age. a), b) and c) Anterior, lateral and posterior views. Note the striking pectus carinatum, the acromesomelic shortness, the prominent abdomen and the dolichocephaly with prominent forehead. d) Close-up of the short and chubby hands. e) The feet with prominent heels and short 2nd toes.

descended. The forearms and hands were short; there were simian creases and clinodactyly of the 5th fingers. The lower limbs were also short, mainly in the acromesomelic segments, and in both feet bilateral brachydactyly of the 2nd toe and a prominent heel were observed (Fig. 2).

Results of laboratory studies including blood cell count, urinalysis, blood and urine chemistries, serum proteins by electrophoresis, liver and thyroid function tests, screening tests for metabolic defects (ferric chloride, DNPH, Benedict's, nitroprusside-cyanide, mucopolysaccharides by turbidometric method), urinary excretion of α-amino nitrogen, plasma aminogram (using a Beckman amino acid analyzer model 120-C), X-chromatin, and karyotype were normal.

Roentgenograms showed various abnormalities. The skull showed craniofacial disproportion and frontal prominences, mild separation of the sutures (more evident in the coronal sutures) and the base was short with a J-shaped sella (Fig. 3). The thorax showed pectus carinatum with chondrocostal enlargement; the sternum was short. The axial skeleton showed generalized platyspondyly and the 12th dorsal vertebral body had a "bullet" shape, the intervertebral spaces were in-

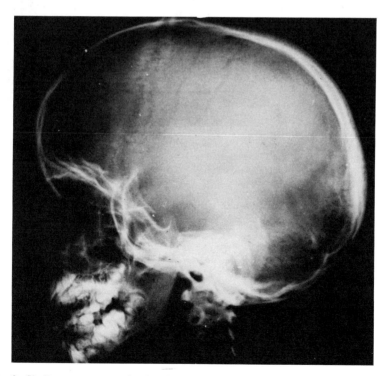

Fig. 3. Skull roentgenogram showing the craniofacial disproportion and dolichocephaly.

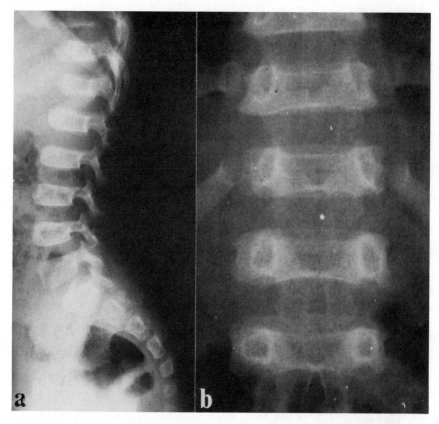

Fig. 4. a) Lateral projection of the spine showing the generalized platyspondyly and the "bullet" morphology of the 12th vertebral body. b) Partial AP projection of the spine with an apparently normal interpediculate distance.

Fig. 5. X-ray film of the pelvis.

Fig. 6. X-ray film of right arm. The tubular bones are thick; the forearm is very short and the ossification nucleus of the radius is absent.

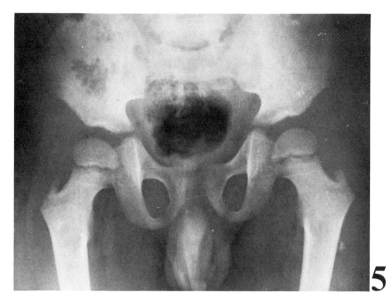

5

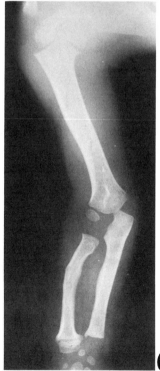

6

creased, and moderate dorsal kyphosis and lumbar lordosis were also observed (Fig. 4). The pelvis was short due to a diminished height of the ilia; the acetabular angle, and the proximal ossification center of the femur were normal (Fig. 5). The bones of the upper limbs were short and wide with moderately irregular metaphyses (Fig. 6). The shortness of the bones was more apparent in the mesomelic portions. The metacarpals and the phalanges were short, broad and osteoporotic (Fig. 7a). The feet were short, broad, and osteoporotic (Fig. 7b). A relative shortness of the 2nd metatarsal was also observed. In the lower limbs, shortness and widening of the long bones, more evident in the mesomelic portion, were observed (Fig. 8).

Progress

At 5½ years the clinical picture has not changed. The length is 80.5 cm, the weight is 12.2 kg. The cephalic, thoracic, and abdominal circumferences are 51, 50, and 52, respectively. The U/L segment ratio is 1.45 (47.7/32.8).

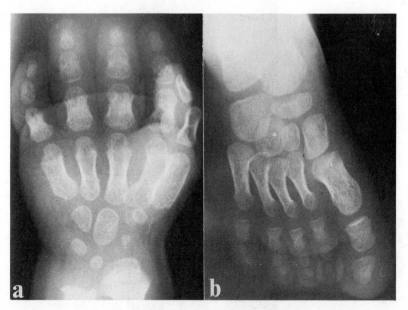

Fig. 7. a) The hand bones are osteoporotic, short and wide. b) The feet bones also show osteoporosis and shortness. The 2nd metacarpal relative shortening can be noticed.

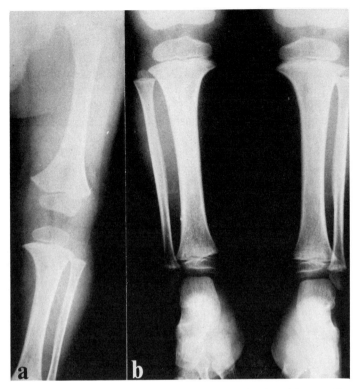

Fig. 8. a) General view of the left leg. b) The tibia and the fibula are short and broad.

Family Data

The parents (*III-9* and *III-10*, Fig. 1) are first cousins and were 24 (father) and 20 (mother) yr old at the birth of the propositus. The parents and their two other children (*IV-15* and *IV-16*) are all normal. The mother has had two spontaneous first trimester abortions. There was no history of a similar pattern of anomalies in 8 paternal and 6 maternal aunts and uncles, in 14 paternal cousins, or in ancestors of previous generations.

DISCUSSION

The syndrome observed in this patient consists mainly of dwarfism, craniofacial disproportion with prominent forehead, short neck and trunk with pectus carinatum and platyspondyly, protuberant abdomen with hepatosplenomegaly (probably due to a reduced thoracic volume), acromesomelic shortness, bilateral simian creases, short feet with brachydactyly of the 2nd toe, and prominent heels. With respect to the differential diagnosis, the pertinent forms of osteochondrodysplastic dwarfism were considered [2–5]. Although the face does not have a gross resemblance to achondroplasia the roentgenologic cranial picture is very similar to that disorder [6]. However, the acromesomelic shortness and the platyspondyly exclude the diagnosis of achondroplasia in the present case. Hypochondroplasia was also ruled out [7].

Regarding the skletal dysplasias which show generalized platyspondyly [8], the following entities were considered: a) Spondyloepiphyseal dysplasia congenita [9] which presents pectus carinatum, normal-sized hands and feet, and severe skeletal deformities; b) spondyloepiphyseal dysplasia tarda [10] which shows (besides the late onset of the disorder) small iliac and long pubic and ischial bones; c) brachyolmia [8] which presents only short trunk; d) Kozlowski spondylo-metaphyseal dysostosis [11]; Morquio disease [2] which shows normal-sized limbs; f) Dyggve-Melchior-Clausen disease [12] in which short hands are present, but characterized by irregular epiphysometaphyseal ossification and short trunk dwarfism; g) metatropic dwarfism [13]; and h) Kniest disease [14] which is characterized by small thorax, early platyspondyly and late kyphoscoliosis, severe metaphyseal flaring, and epiphyseal irregularities.

The clinical and radiologic features of the syndrome observed in the patient, plus the parental consanguinity, strongly suggest a genetic etiology, probably mendelian autosomal recessive. This patient was first misdiagnosed as having achondroplasia; To avoid misdiagnosis when studying individuals with short-limb dwarfism, we suggest the patient be checked for platyspondyly, the most typical feature in this syndrome.

SUMMARY

An infant with a distinct set of skeletal anomalies was studied. The patient's main phenotypic features were short-limb dwarfism, craniofacial disproportion with prominent forehead, short neck and trunk with pectus carinatum, and platyspondyly, protuberant abdomen, acromesomelic shortness of limbs, bilateral palm simian crease, short feet with brachydactyly of the 2nd toe, and prominent heels. Differential diagnosis suggests that the case described had a previously unrecognized skeletal dysplasia. The fact that the parents were first cousins suggests a genetic, probably autosomal recessive etiology.

REFERENCES

1. Ramos-Galván R: Somatometría pediátrica. Estudio semilongitudinal en ninos de la Ciudad de México. Arch Inv Med (Mex) 6:83, 1975.
2. McKusick VA: "Heritable Disorders of Connective Tissue." St Louis: CV Mosby, 1972.

3. Bergsma D (ed): "Birth Defects Atlas and Compendium." Baltimore: Williams & Wilkins for The National Foundation–March of Dimes, 1973.
4. Spranger JW, Langer LO, Wiedemann HR: "Bone Dysplasias. An Atlas of Constitutional Disorders of Skeletal Development." Philadelphia: WB Saunders, 1974.
5. McKusick VA: "Mendelian Inheritance in Man," 4th Ed. Baltimore: Johns Hopkins Press, 1975.
6. Ponseti JV: Skeletal growth in achrondroplasia. J Bone Joint Surg 52A:701, 1970.
7. Walker BA, Murdoch L, McKusick VA, Langer LP, Beals RK: Hypochondroplasia. Am J Dis Child 122:95, 1971.
8. Maroteaux P: Spondyloepiphyseal dysplasias and metatropic dwarfism. In Bergsma D (ed): Part IV. "Skeletal Dysplasias." White Plains: The National Foundation–March of Dimes, BD:OAS V(4):35, 1969.
9. Spranger J, Langer LO: Spondyloepiphyseal dysplasia congenita. Radiology 94:313, 1970.
10. Maroteaux P, Lamy M, Bernard J: La dysplasie spondyloepiphysaire tardive. Nouv Presse Med 65:1205, 1957.
11. Kozlowski K, Maroteaux P, Spranger J: La dystostose spondylométaphysaire. Nouv Presse Med 75:2769, 1967.
12. Dyggve HV, Melchior JC, Clausen J: Morquio-Ullrich's disease, an inborn error of metabolism? Arch Dis Child 37:525, 1962.
13. Maroteaux P, Spranger JW, Wiedemann H-R: Der metatropische zwergwuchs. Arch Kinderheilkd 173:211, 1966;
14. Maroteaux P, Spranger J: La maladie de Kniest. Arch Fr Pediatr 30:735, 1973.

An Unusual Familial Spondyloepiphyseal Dysplasia: "Spondyloperipheral Dysplasia"

Thaddeus E. Kelly, MD, PhD, Jack R. Lichtenstein, MD, and John P. Dorst, MD

INTRODUCTION

The spondyloepiphyseal dysplasias have been differentiated on the basis of the time of onset and the pattern of vertebral and peripheral involvement [1]. In those with delayed onset, or the tarda forms, peripheral involvement with only localized involvement of the vertebral column is characteristic of the multiple epiphyseal dysplasias, while generalized platyspondyly with hip involvement has been considered characteristic of the spondyloepiphyseal dysplasias. Distinction between the entities may at times be ill-defined [2]. An unusual skeletal dysplasia, consisting of generalized platyspondyly, narrowing of the joint spaces in the elbows, wrists, and hips, and shortening of the forearm and small tubular bones will be reported in this article.

CASE REPORTS

Case 1. A 60-yr-old white male has been short all his life. He had had intermittent bilateral hip pain since 21 yr of age and recently developed pain in his elbows. He had had mild hypertension and a stroke. His parents were of normal stature (Fig. 1). His brother and sister and eight nieces and nephews were all of normal height. He was married to his maternal first cousin and has two children of similar habitus.

Physical examination in 1975 showed him to be a short-limbed dwarf with a normal facies and skull. His height was 142 cm, span 127 cm, and upper to lower ratio, 1.12 (Fig. 2). He had marked shortness of the forearms and bilaterally

Birth Defects: Original Article Series, Volume XIII, Number 3B, pages 149—165

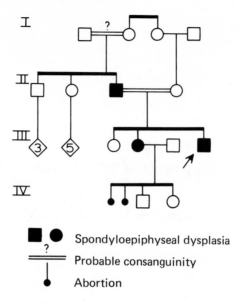

Fig. 1. Pedigree consistent with autosomal dominant or recessive inheritance.

absent ulnar styloid processes. He could not fully extend his elbows. He had brachydactyly of the hands and feet, coxa vara, and walked with a waddling gait.

Case 2. The 31-yr-old daughter of *Case 1* was the product of a normal pregnancy and was not noticed to be small until age 4 years. She had pain in her left knee and left hip, and walked with a limp since 15 years. At 18 years, radiographs showed absence of the distal left ulna but not the right, dorsal kyphosis, and vertebral irregularities diagnosed as Scheuermann disease.

Her two children were delivered by cesarean section and were clinically and radiographically unaffected.

Physical examination in 1975 showed a short-limbed dwarf, with a normal facies and skull (Fig. 3). Her height was 141 cm, span 142 cm, and upper to lower ratio, 0.73. She had mild brachydactyly of the hands. The left ulnar styloid was not palpable, but was palpable on the right. She could fully extend her elbows. Increased lumbar lordosis and moderate dorsal kyphosis were noted. There was decreased abduction of the left hip. The 3rd, 4th, and 5th toes were short bilaterally.

Case 3. The 30-yr-old son of *Case 1* was the product of a normal pregnancy and has been small since early childhood. He denied arthralgias. He was

Fig. 2. *Case 1* at 60 years.

Fig. 3. *Case 2* at 31 years.

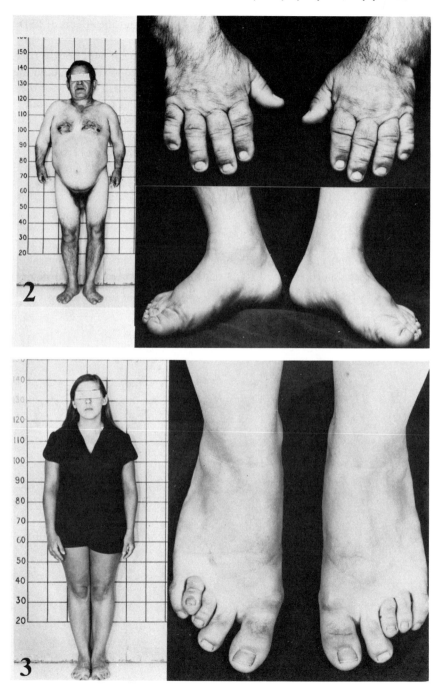

the propositus in this family and initially consulted us about the effects of LSD on chromosomes.

Physical examination in 1975 showed a short-limbed dwarf with normal facies (Fig. 4). His height was 158 cm, span 130 cm, and upper to lower ratio, 0.96. He had marked limitation of extension at the elbows. He had brachydactyly of the fingers and toes, trident hands, and hyperextensibility of his fingers. Increased lumbar lordosis was observed. There was a full range of motion at the hips.

Chest, eyes, teeth, and intelligence were normal in these cases.

Results of routine laboratory studies in *Cases 2* and *3,* including hematocrit, calcium, phosphorus, alkaline phosphatase, and urinary amino acid chromatography and mucopolysaccharide spot test were normal.

ROENTGENOLOGIC FINDINGS

Case 1

Right upper limb (Fig. 5): All bones are short, and the shortness increases distally acromelic shortness. A) Lateral view of the elbow and B) frontal view

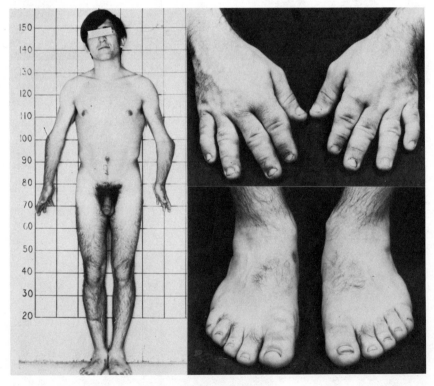

Fig. 4. *Case 3* at 30 years.

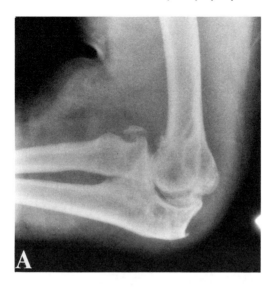

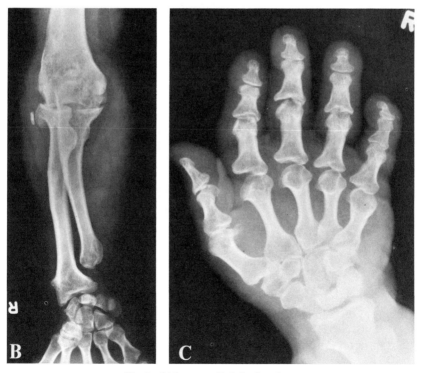

Fig. 5. Right upper limb in *Case 1*.

of the forearm show greatly deformed ends of the bones, with a mushroom-shaped radial head that is slightly anteriorly subluxated with anterior and lateral accessory ossicles and an unusually prominent radial tuberosity. The distal end of the ulnar is 2 cm short of the radius at the wrist. C) All of the metacarpals and phalanges are greatly shortened, with most severe involvement of the distal phalanges; the 5th distal phalanx is also bowed as in the Kirner deformity. The bases of the middle and proximal phalanges are concave, suggesting that the previous epiphyses were cone shaped, and the interphalangeal joints are quite narrow. The carpus, although actually small, is less affected and appears relatively large.

Spine (Fig. 6): There is generalized platyspondyly, greatest in the midthoracic spine and minimal in the cervical spine, and moderate degenerative joint

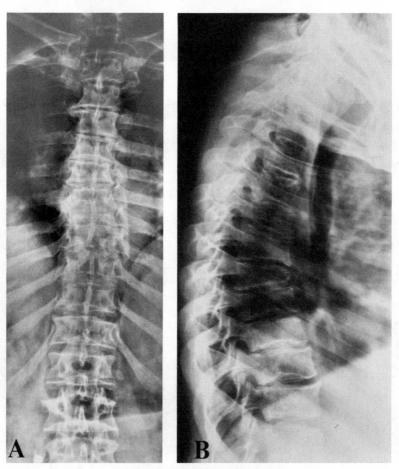

Fig. 6. Spine in *Case 1.*

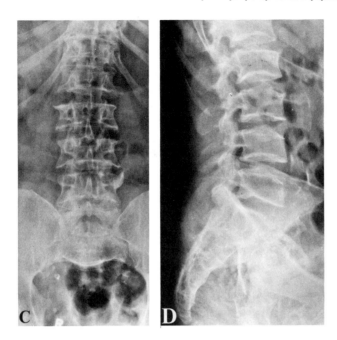

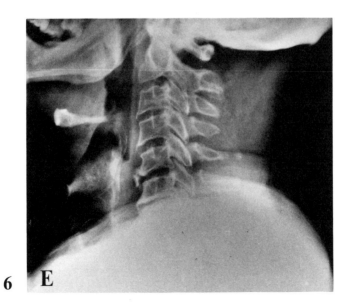

6

disease. In the thoracic spine the intervertebral disks are narrow and the superior and inferior surfaces of the vertebral bodies are moderately irregular, while in the lumbar spine they form arcs.

Pelvis and hips (Fig. 7): The pelvis is tilted somewhat forward and femoral necks are in varus. The femoral heads are large and irregular with cyst-like radiolucencies and eburnated surfaces. The joint cartilage is narrow, particularly on the right side.

Feet (Fig. 8): Short and wide feet show moderate foreshortening of the tarsus and great foreshortening of the metatarsals and phalanges. The interphalangeal joints are quite narrow.

Case 2

Hands (Fig. 9): The acromelic shortness is far less severe than in the other two patients, and the ends of the long bones are more normally formed. The left, but not the right, ulna is foreshortened distally, and the left 5th metacarpal is considerably more foreshortened than the right. Phalanges are short, particularly the

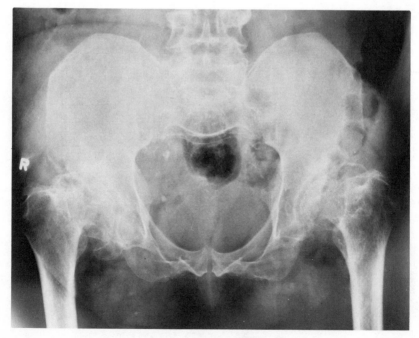

Fig. 7. Pelvis and hips in *Case 1*.

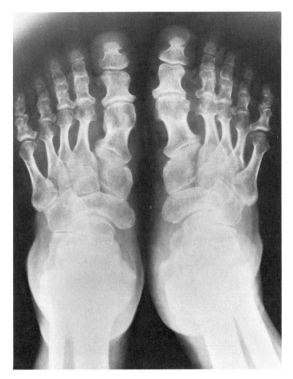

Fig. 8. Feet in *Case 1*.

middle phalanges, with slightly concave bases and extremely narrow interphalangeal joint cartilages. There is slight bowing of the distal phalanges of the little fingers.

Spine (Fig. 10): The platyspondyly is slightly less severe than in the other two patients. A) The cervical spine is almost normal. B) In the thoracic spine there is increased kyphosis with considerable narrowing of the intervertebral disks and moderate irregularity of the superior and inferior surfaces of the vertebral bodies. C) and D) In the lumbar spine, the changes are much less pronounced — minimal platyspondyly, with mild irregularity of the end plates and no narrowing of the intervertebral disks. Yet the lower spinal canal is narrow since the pedicles ar relatively short, and there is almost no widening of the lower lumbar and upper sacral interpediculate spaces.

Pelvis and lateral film of hip (Fig. 11): There is moderately severe coxa valga, with shallow acetabular cavities and mild lateral subluxation of the femoral heads, which contain cyst-like radiolucencies with thin sclerotic margins. The femurs,

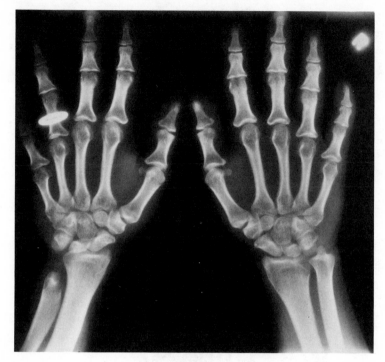

Fig. 9. Hands in *Case 2*.

tibias, and fibulas (not illustrated) are slightly short but otherwise almost normal, but there is moderate foreshortening of the feet with especially short 3rd and 4th metatarsals.

Case 3

Upper limb (Fig. 12): A) Upper limb bones show acromelic shortening and considerable deformity and irregularity of their ends, most striking at the elbow, where there is eburnation and narrowing of joint cartilage. B) The ulna is 3 cm short of the radius at the wrist. C) All bones of the wrist and hand are foreshortened, with least involvement of the first three metacarpals. The bases of the proximal and middle phalanges are concave, suggesting that the previous epiphyses were cone shaped. The joint cartilages are thin.

Spine (Fig. 13): There is generalized platyspondyly. A) Minimal in the cervical spine, and B) greatest in the thoracic spine. In the thoracic spine, intervertebral disks are narrow and the surfaces of the vertebral bodies are irregular and tend to be curved. C) In the lumbar spine there is considerably less widening of

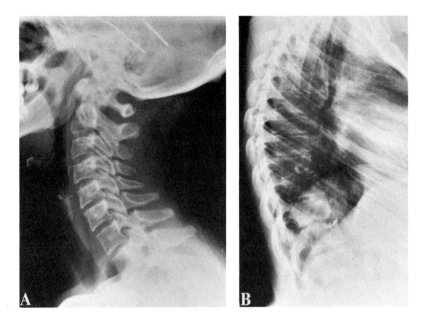

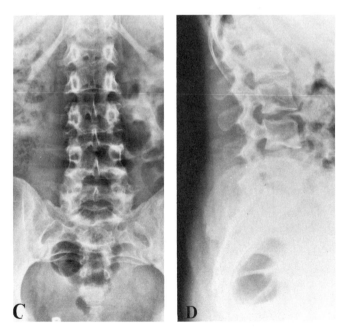

Fig. 10. Spine in *Case 2*.

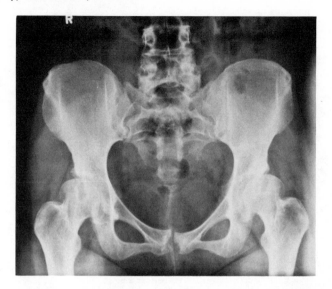

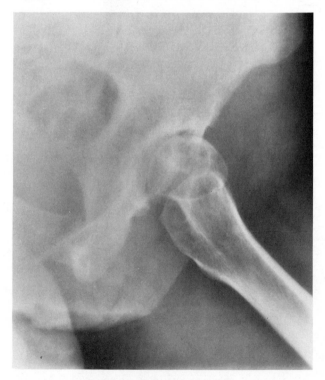

Fig. 11. Pelvis and hip in *Case 2*.

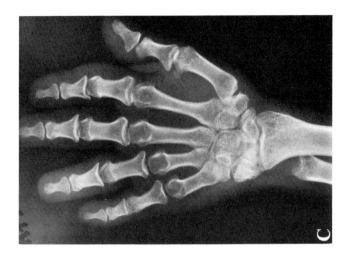

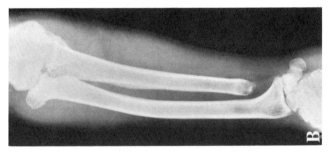

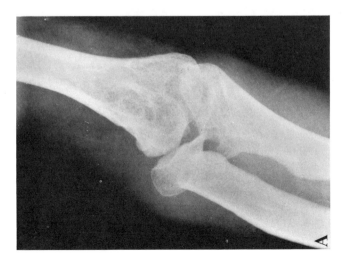

Fig. 12. Upper limb in *Case 3.*

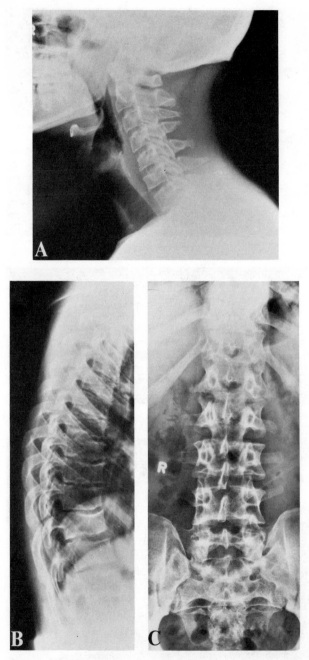

Fig. 13. Spine in *Case 3*.

the lower lumbar and upper sacral interpediculate spaces than normal. Moreover, the lateral roentgenogram (not reproduced) shows short pedicles, so that the lower lumbar spine canal is relatively narrow.

Pelvis and hips (Fig. 14): There is a somewhat narrow pelvis with relatively shallow acetabular cavities and hips in mild valgus. The joint cartilage is narrow superiorly, with eburnation of the femoral heads and acetabular roofs, and cyst-like radiolucencies in the femoral heads.

Feet (Fig. 15): The feet are short and wide due to foreshortening of all bones. Interphalangeal joint cartilages are relatively narrow.

DISCUSSION

Although there is vertical transmission of this condition, there is probable consanguinity in *Generation I* and definite consanguinity in *Generation II*. The pedigree in this family is therefore compatible with either autosomal dominant or autosomal recessive inheritance. The unaffected son in *Generation IV*, the affected son, and the affected daughter in *Generation III* eliminated the possibility of X-linked inheritance.

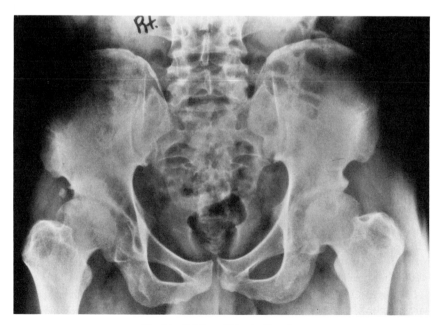

Fig. 14. Pelvis and hips in *Case 3*.

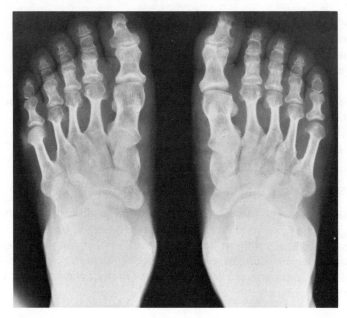

Fig. 15. Feet in *Case 3*.

Since abnormalities were not recognized in *Case 2* until she was age 4 yr, it is probable that the changes in this disorder do not occur until childhood. The peripheral changes of narrowing of the joints of the forearm and hips and shortening of the forearm and small tubular bones could be compatible with multiple epiphyseal dysplasia; however, the generalized vertebral changes are not seen in that disorder [1]. The platyspondyly is not as severe as is commonly seen in X-linked spondyloepiphyseal dysplasia tarda, and peripheral changes are usually absent in that condition [3, 7, 8]. Platyspondyly and peripheral changes have been described in the dominantly inherited form of spondyloepiphyseal dysplasia tarda. Rubin [2] described a family with vertebral pelvic and peripheral radiologic changes (Figs. 7 and 9, 7.10—7.14 in Rubin's book), similar to this family and with autosomal dominant inheritance, as spondyloepiphyseal dysplasia tarda. In pseudoachondroplastic dysplasia (formerly pseudoachondroplastic type of spondyloepiphyseal dysplasia, McKusick and Scott, 1971) the dwarfism is much more severe than in this family, and is rhizomelic [4]. Other reports have emphasized the difficulties in classifying cases of apparent multiple epiphyseal dysplasia with generalized vertebral involvement [2, 5, 6].

There are other reports of skeletal dysplasia with dwarfism and vertebral and peripheral changes which can be distinguished from that described here. Robinow [10] described three of seven female sibs by normal parents with "spondylo-epiphyseal dysplasia with peripheral dysostosis." The radiographs showed massive, rectangular mandibles, mild thoracolumbar platyspondyly, thick, short humeri with a midshaft bulge and small carpals and short metacarpals. Nance and Sweeney [11] described a recessively inherited chondrodystrophy which combined features of achondroplasia, pseudoachondroplasia and diastrophic dwarfism. Acromesomelic dwarfism described by Maroteaux et al [12] differs from the disorder described here by more striking dwarfism, less severe vertebral and pelvic changes, radial, rather than ulnar hypoplasia, and striking mesomelia.

A distinctive finding in the cases reported here was shortening of the distal ulna. This finding has also been reported in multiple exostoses and as an extreme normal variant [9]. These diagnoses are not tenable in the cases in this report. Our cases may be a variant of multiple epiphyseal dysplasia or a distinct form of spondyloepiphyseal dysplasia which we term "spondyloperipheral dysplasia."

REFERENCES

1. Maroteaux P: Spondyloepiphyseal dysplasias and metatropic dwarfism. In (Bergsma D, ed): Part IV. "Skeletal Dysplasias." New York: The National Foundation – March of Dimes, BD:OAS V(4):35–44, 1969.
2. Rubin P: "Dynamic Classification of Bone Dysplasias." Chicago: Year Book Medical Publishers, 1964, pp 85–159.
3. Langer LO Jr: Spondyloepiphyseal dysplasia tarda. Radiology 82:833, 1965.
4. Hall JG, Dorst JP: Pseudoachondroplastic SED, recessive Maroteaux-Lamy type. In "Skeletal Dysplasias." op cit pp 254–259.
5. Hobaek A: "Problems of Hereditary Chondrodysplasia." Oslo: Oslo University Press, 1961.
6. Felman AH: Multiple epiphyseal dysplasia. Cases with unusual vertebral involvement. Radiology 93:119 1969.
7. Solomon L: Bone growth in diaphyseal dysplasias. J Bone Joint Surg 43B:700–716, 1961.
8. Hultén O: Uber anatomische Variationen der handgelenkknochen. Acta Radiol 9:155–167, 1928.
9. Spranger JW, Langer LO, Wiedemann HR: "Bone Dysplasias: An Atlas of Constitutional Disorders of Skeletal Development." Philadelphia: WB Saunders, 1974.
10. Robinow M: A spondyloepiphyseal dysplasia with peripheral dysostosis. In Bergsma D (ed): "Clinical Cytogenetics and Genetics." Miami: Symposia Specialists for The National Foundation–March of Dimes, BD:OAS X (9):67–73, 1974.
11. Nance WE, Sweeney A: "A Recessively Inherited Chondrodystrophy." Bergsma D (ed): New York: The National Foundation–March of Dimes, BD:OAS VI (4):25–27, 1970.
12. Maroteaux P, Martinelli B, Campailla E: Le nanisme acromesomelique. Presse Med 79:1839–1842, 1971.

Duplication 11 (q21 to 23→qter) Syndrome*

Uta Francke, MD, Felice Weber, MD, Robert S. Sparkes, MD,
Philip D. Mattson, MD, and John Mann, MD

The delineation of clinical syndromes associated with duplications of certain chromosome regions—as opposed to whole extra chromosomes or chromosome arms—is more difficult because of variations in the extent of the duplicated chromosome region in different families, and because in cases with inherited translocations the associated monosomies may involve completely different chromosomal regions. Nevertheless, it appears that a syndrome of congenital abnormalities, all of which are individually nonspecific, is produced by duplication of the distal one-third to one-half of the long arm of chromosome 11 which may allow recognition of the syndrome on a clinical basis.

In this article we discuss three patients from unrelated families with different reciprocal translocations involving 11q. Each pedigree contains an additional individual who appeared to have the clinical syndrome, but could not be studied.

CASE REPORTS

Patient 1

The propositus was born after a 40-week uncomplicated pregnancy to a 23-year-old primigravida. Delivery was vaginal with manual change from an occipitoposterior to an occipitoanterior position. The umbilical cord was wrapped three times around his neck. Apgar scores were 6 and 8. He weighed

*This work was supported by research grants GM-21110, GM-17702, and HD-05615 from the United States Public Health Service, by a grant from the National Foundation-March of Dimes, and by the San Diego Regional Center for the Developmentally Disabled.

Birth Defects: Original Article Series, Volume XIII, Number 3B, pages 167—186
© 1977 The National Foundation

2,280 gm and was 48 cm long. The newborn was noted to have abnormalities of the head, a small pharynx, a small penis (1 cm), varus deformity of the feet, a heart murmur, and increased cardiac size. He had to be gavage fed because of sucking and swallowing difficulties. When discharged from the hospital at 13 days, he had gained weight and was in stable condition.

At 5 months, his length was 63.5 cm (10th percentile) and his weight was 7 kg (50th percentile) (Fig. 1). The head was small (occipitofrontal circumference 39.5 cm, below 3rd percentile) and asymmetric, tilted to the right and turned to the left. The anterior fontanel was fibrous and measured 1 cm X 1 cm; the metopic suture was prominent. There was very fine sparse blond hair which extended to the right cheek. The scalp veins were prominent.

He had marked hypotelorism with an inner canthal distance of 1.8 cm, an outer canthal distance of 6.5 cm, and interpupillary distance of 3.6 cm. Eye examination was normal except for variable alternating esotropia. The face was asymmetric probably secondary to the torticollis. The nose was short and the philtrum elongated. The palate was high and narrow due to double alveolar ridge. The tongue was tied by a short frenulum. The mandible was short, resulting in a retracted lower lip and a dimple on the receding chin. The auricles were appa-

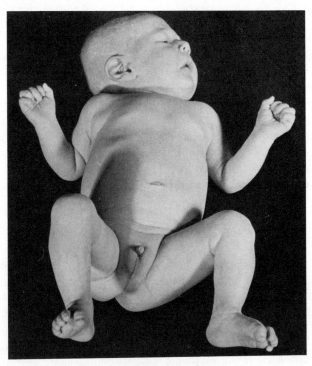

Fig. 1. *Patient 1* at 5 months.

rently low set and posteriorly rotated, 4.8 cm long, and shaped unequally.

The chest circumference was 44 cm with an internipple distance of 9 cm. The nipples were hypoplastic and inverted. A grade 3/6 holosystolic murmur was audible over the entire precordium. Aside from slight perioral cyanosis with crying, there was no sign of cardiac decompensation.

The penis which had been very small at birth now measured 4 cm as a result of local treatment with testosterone cream (Fig. 2). Both testicles, 1.2 cm in length, were present in a hypoplastic scrotum. There was a blind pilonidal dimple.

Abduction was limited in both hips, and creases on the thighs were asymmetric. The feet were in varus position. Elevation of both arms was limited. Elbows were flexed and fists were clenched. The hand lengths were 7.5 cm, and the feet 8.0 cm.

The skin was slightly mottled. A capillary hemangioma was noted in the occipital region. There were dimples at both elbows. Palmar and plantar creases were not unusual. Fingertip patterns consisted of arches on both thumbs and

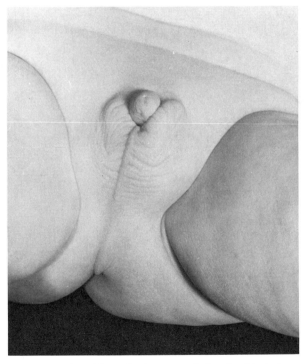

Fig. 2. *Patient 1.* Micropenis and hypoplastic scrotum before local testosterone treatment.

index fingers and ulnar loops on the remaining fingers, while both parents had 10 ulnar loops. The digital palmar "a" triradius at the base of both 2nd digits was displaced radically.

Deep tendon reflexes were equal and normoactive, Babinski reflexes were absent, Moro and neck righting reflexes were still present. General muscle tone was decreased except for the lower limbs where it was variable and occasionally increased. In prone position he could lift his head up briefly and roll to the side. Head control was poor. He did not bear weight on his legs. He did not follow objects across the midline and did not smile spontaneously.

The child received physical therapy and was enrolled in an infant stimulation program. He had multiple operations for inguinal hernias, for dislocation of the right hip, and for placement of polyethylene tubes to drain his middle ears. The torticollis was treated by manual stretching. Radiologic examination of his cervical spine did not disclose any definite abnormalities. Chest films taken in the neonatal period and later consistently showed cardiomegaly and incomplete development of the right clavicle with lack of fusion between the lateral and the medial portion (Fig. 3). A lateral skull film and intravenous pyelogram were normal. The acetabulas were shallow on hip radiographs.

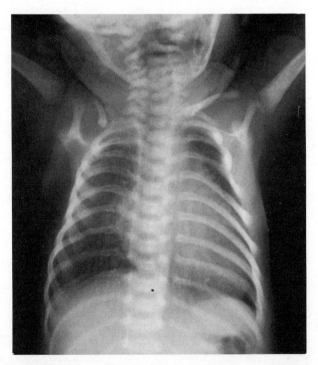

Fig. 3. *Patient 1.* Chest radiograph. Note defect of right clavicle and cardiomegaly.

At 17 months, his length was 78 cm (10th percentile) with an upper to lower segment ratio of 1.5. Head circumference was 42.8 cm (below 3rd percentile). In addition to the dysmorphic findings noted earlier, there were intermittent nystagmus and more pronounced hypoplasia of the right side of the face. The maxilla was prominent and the philtrum was long with a distinctive Cupid's bow. He was retracting the lower lip and sucking on it (Fig. 4). No teeth had erupted yet, although rudimentary tooth buds were present on radiographs of mandible and maxilla. There was a loud systolic cardiac murmur; the liver was palpable 2 cm below the right costal margin. He was able to roll over, but unable to sit. He did not reach out for objects, nor did he transfer objects from one hand to the other. There were stereotypic turning movements of his hands in bilateral synchrony with wrists in extension and fingers spread. He responded to sound and to visual stimuli. Electroencephalographic audiometry indicated a mild to moderate hearing loss in the high frequency range. Echocardiography results were consistent with an endocardial cushion defect.

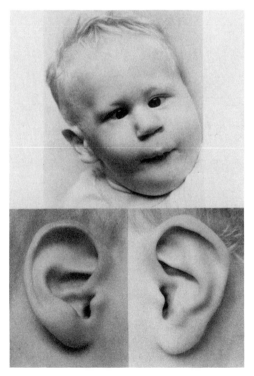

Fig. 4. *Patient 1* at 17 months. Note facial asymmetry, hypotelorism, long philtrum, and short mandible with retracted lower lip.

Chromosome studies. All metaphases analyzed with trypsin-Giemsa banding from the propositus' blood and fibroblast cultures showed a male karyotype with an elongated chromosome 6 (46,XY,6q+) (Fig. 5a). A small amount of faintly staining chromosome material had been translocated to the end of the long arm of a chromosome 6. A balanced and presumably reciprocal translocation—46,XX,t(6;11) (q27;q2300)—was identified in the patient's mother and permitted the definition of the extra material present in the patient as region 11q2300→11qter; ie the distal third of the long arm of chromosome 11 (Fig. 5b). The same balanced t(6;11) translocation was found in the maternal grandfather (*II-2*) and in a maternal uncle (*III-1*) (Fig. 6).

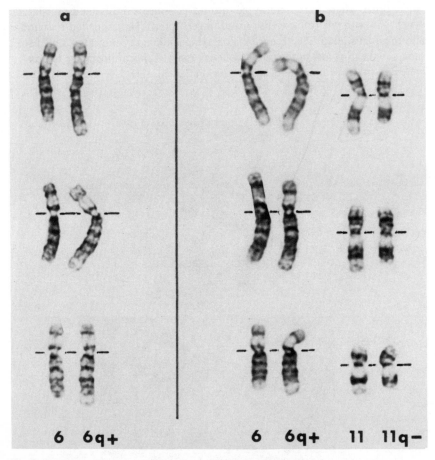

6   6q+   6   6q+   11   11q—

Fig. 5. Partial karyotypes with G-banding. a) Three chromosome pairs 6 from *Patient 1* showing the abnormal chromosome 6q+, all other chromosomes were normal; karyotype designation is 46,XY,6q+. b) Three sets of chromosome pairs 6 and 11 from balanced translocation heterozygote; karyotype designation is 46,XX, t(6;11) (q27;q2300) (For banded diagram of chromosome 11 see Fig. 12).

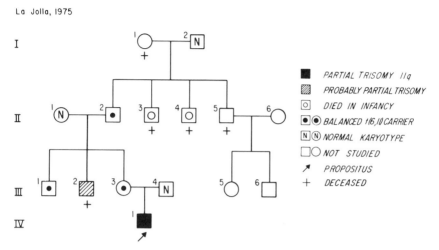

La Jolla, 1975

Fig. 6. Pedigree. The propositus (*IV-1*) is *Patient 1* of this article.

Another maternal uncle, (*III-2*), who was severely retarded and died at 9 yr, had resembled our patient in many aspects. He was born with a small penis and short tongue frenulum. On family photographs one can distinguish his small head, hypotelorism, low-set ears, short nose and long philtrum, and receding chin with dimple. Abnormalities noted at autopsy included decreased brain size with thickened areas of the dura. Microscopic sections of the brain showed multiple areas of scarring. The pituitary gland had a decreased number of cells. There were no cardiac or renal abnormalities. The CNS findings taken together with a history of "meningitis" at 2 years of age were thought to be responsible for the child's retardation. However, his psychomotor development had been slow since birth. We consider it more likely that he had inherited the 6q+ chromosome from his father, and thus had the 11q duplication syndrome.

Gene marker studies. The propositus and both parents were typed for the following blood groups, red cell enzymes, and serum proteins: ABO, Le, Rh, Duffy, MNSs, Lu, Kell, Kp, Kidd, P1, AK, 6-PGD, ADA, PGM1, AcP1, haptoglobin, alpha1-antitrypsin, esterase D, amylase, and hemoglobin. The results were not informative for gene localization.

Patient 2

The proband was born after a term uncomplicated pregnancy to a 20-yr-old primigravida. She weighed 2,600 gm and was 49 cm long. Her head circumference was 32.5 cm. She did not breathe spontaneously and was cyanotic. Hypoplastic mandible and cleft soft palate led to the diagnosis of Pierre-Robin syndrome. The left hip was dislocated. During her hospital course she had feeding difficulties and cyanotic episodes due to upper airway obstruction by the relatively large tongue. A heart murmur was noted at 2 weeks. The heart was enlarged on roentgenograms and EKG showed right axis deviation and right ventricular hypertrophy. A tracheostomy was performed at 5 weeks because of continued airway obstruction. She died shortly afterwards from cardiac arrest.

A postmortem examination revealed hypoplasia of the mandible and cleft palate, glossoptosis, marked mediastinal emphysema, atelectasis of both lungs, extensive mononuclear infiltration of alveoli, interatrial septal defect, agenesis of the right kidney, hypertrophy of the left kidney, agenesis of the right fallopian tube, bilateral congenital dislocation of hips, bilateral inguinal hernias, agenesis of the corpus callosum, and hypoplasia of vermis of cerebellum. It was thought that the marked mediastinal emphysema was a major factor leading to death and probably a consequence of air entering through the tracheostomy wound. At the time of autopsy, the patient weighed 2,770 gm and measured 46 cm in length.

Chromosome studies with standard staining showed a 46,XX,Bq+ karyotype. Cytogenetic analysis was performed on all available family members. The patient's mother was found to have an identical Bq+ chromosome and, in addition, a shortened, unusually metacentric C-group chromosome: 46,XX,t(Bq+;Cq–). The apparently balanced translocation was inherited from the maternal grandmother, and was also present in a maternal uncle and aunt. Autoradiographic analysis identified the B-group chromosome involved as a number 4. When Q-banding became available, a balanced translocation carrier was restudied and the translocation was identified as balanced t(4q+;11q–). The proposita was diagnosed, in retrospect, as the first case of partial trisomy for the distal long arm of chromosome 11 [1]. G-banding has since confirmed these results and has permitted localization of the break points: t(4;11) (q35;q23.1) (Fig. 7).

The pedigree is shown in Figure 8. No spontaneous abortions were reported among the offspring of the four balanced translocation carriers. A first cousin of our proposita *(III-4)* was identified as having a 46,XY,4q+ karyotype indicating 11q duplication (Fig. 7a). He was known to be developmentally retarded, but was subsequently lost to follow-up and could not be examined.

Fig. 7. *Patient 2.* G-banded karyotypes of family members. a) 46,XY,4q+ or 46,XY,der (4) t(4;11) (q35;q23.1), karyotype of individual *III-4* with partial trisomy 11q. Arrow indicates abnormal chromosome 4q+. b) Karyotype of balanced translocation heterozgote *II-3*: 46,XX,t(4;11) (q35;q23.1). Arrows indicate translocation chromosomes.

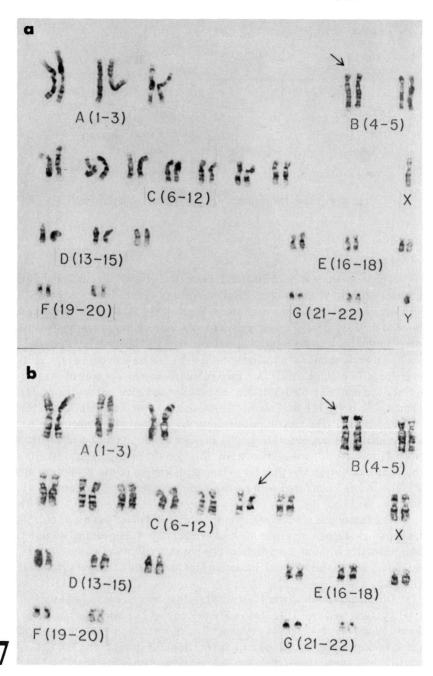

a

A (1–3)

B (4–5)

C (6–12)

X

D (13–15)

E (16–18)

F (19–20)

G (21–22)

Y

b

A (1–3)

B (4–5)

C (6–12)

X

D (13–15)

E (16–18)

F (19–20)

G (21–22)

7

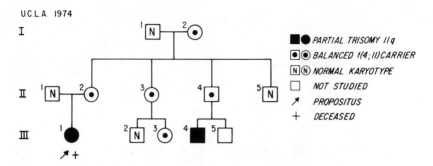

UCLA. 1974

■● PARTIAL TRISOMY 11q
⊡⊙ BALANCED t(4;11)CARRIER
Ⓝℕ NORMAL KARYOTYPE
☐ NOT STUDIED
↗ PROPOSITUS
+ DECEASED

Fig. 8. Pedigree. The proposita *(III-1)* is *Patient 2* of this article.

Patient 3

The proposita was born by breech delivery after a 39-week uncomplicated pregnancy to a 30-yr-old mother. Fetal movements were described as weak. The cord was wrapped around the neck twice. She weighed 2,250 gm at birth and was noted to have apparently low-set ears, a narrow face, micrognathia, webbed neck, low posterior hairline, lax joints, hyperelastic skin, and bilateral hip dysplasia. She had a weak, cat-like cry and congenital heart disease thought to represent an endocardial cushion defect. An intravenous pyelogram was normal. At 1 yr of age, she had marked growth and developmental retardation and was reported by Mann and Rafferty [2] as a case of "Cri-du-chat syndrome combined with partial C-group trisomy." The karyotype interpretation was based on standard staining, sex chromatin studies, autoradiography and Q-banding, and indicated a balanced, probably reciprocal, translocation t(5p+;11q−) in the mother. The proposita's 46,XX,5p+ karyotype was thought to represent deletion of the distal short arm of chromosome 5 combined with partial trisomy for the distal long arm of chromosome 11.

The family was reexamined recently when the patient was 6½ yr old. She has had surgical repair of a right inguinal hernia at age 4. Her cardiac status has remained stable without digitalization. She has suffered from frequent upper respiratory infections. Bilateral dislocated hips have been treated unsuccessfully with casts.

On examination she was 103 cm tall (below 3rd percentile, height age of 4 4/12 yr) and weighed 12 kg (below 3rd percentile). Her head was microcephalic (head circumference 47 cm) and symmetric with a narrow prominent forehead and flat occiput (Fig. 9). Scalp hair was very thin and straight. She had flat supraorbital ridges, short, sparse eyebrows, and sparse eyelashes. The inner canthal distance of 2.7 cm was at the mean, but outer orbital distance of 8.4 cm was signi-

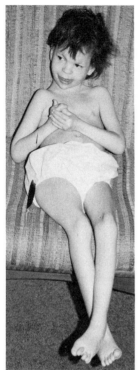
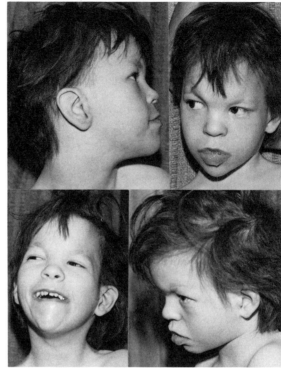

Fig. 9. *Patient 3* at 6 yr of age. (See text for description of dysmorphic features.)

ficantly decreased. Interpupillary distance was 5.3 cm, slightly above the mean. Mann and Rafferty [2] commented previously on the false impression of hypertelorism caused by an abnormally narrow face. There were no abnormal ocular findings. The nose was short and the philtrum elongated. The maxilla appeared hypoplastic. The palate was high with a double alveolar ridge. Teeth were irregular and the lateral incisors were abnormally large. The ears were low set and had prominent antihelices. There was a preauricular tag on the right. The right ear canal was narrower than the left. The neck was normal in size and not webbed. The shoulders were narrow and asymmetric because of incomplete development of the right clavicle which led to "turning in" of the right shoulder. The thorax was bell-shaped and asymmetric due to moderate kyphoscoliosis. Chest circumference was 53 cm, internipple distance 11.5 cm. A low-grade short systolic murmur was audible at the left sternal border. Liver and spleen were not enlarged. There were no masses or hernias, but a scar from a right inguinal hernia repair. The genitalia were normal.

The upper limbs had full range of motion. Fingers and wrists were hyper-extensible. The thumbs were short, broad, and proximally placed. The distal phalanges of all digits were relatively short. Both hips were dislocated and there were flexion contractures at the knees. The patellas were small. The posterior plantar fat pads were thickened.

Dermatoglyphic analysis showed the palmar axial triradii in the t position, wide spaces between the digital palmar triradii a and b at the bases of the 2nd and 3rd fingers, and 5 ulnar loops and 5 whorls on fingertips. Dermal ridges were generally hypoplastic.

The skin was normal except for a capillary hemangioma on the occiput. The musculature was underdeveloped. There were normal deep tendon reflexes and no pathologic reflexes present. The patient was profoundly retarded, unable to sit and roll over. She had poor head control and could not talk. She followed objects with her eyes, but did not reach out. She smiled spontaneously and in response to stimuli.

The patient is the youngest of three sibs; no spontaneous abortions have been reported. A 12-yr-old, phenotypically normal brother is a balanced trans-location carrier (see pedigree in Ref. 2). The second born was a boy who weighed 2,000 gm was 49 cm in length, and died at 1 month from congestive heart failure. He had severe congenital heart disease and a facial appearance and cat-like cry resembling that of the proposita. He also had a highly arched palate, low-set ears, varus deformity of the feet, and a dimple on the chin.

Repeat chromosome analysis on the proposita and her mother have established the points of breakage and rejoining in bands 5p15 and 11q21 (Figs. 10 and 11). The results confirm the previous impression that the translocation is truly reciprocal. The patient is considered to have a deficiency of the distal region of band 5p15 and a duplication of region 11q21→qter. The latter represents a larger portion of 11q than what was duplicated in *Patients 1* and *2*.

DISCUSSION

Unbalanced karyotypes containing a partial duplication of the distal long arm of chromosome 11 have been identified in 3 unrelated patients. They have been compared with 10 previously reported patients [3-9]. As shown in Figure 12, the extent of the duplicated segment varied in different cases. Furthermore, in eight of them, the 11q duplication was associated with a terminal dele-tion of the recipient chromosome involving seven different chromosomal regions (4q, 5p, 6q, 10q, 13q, 17p, 21q). *These deleted segments appear to consist of only a minute part of the telomeric region in most cases.* In *Patient 3,* however, a small 5p− deletion, present in addition to the 11q duplication, could account for the "cat cry" which was a presenting symptom in infancy. Furthermore, there

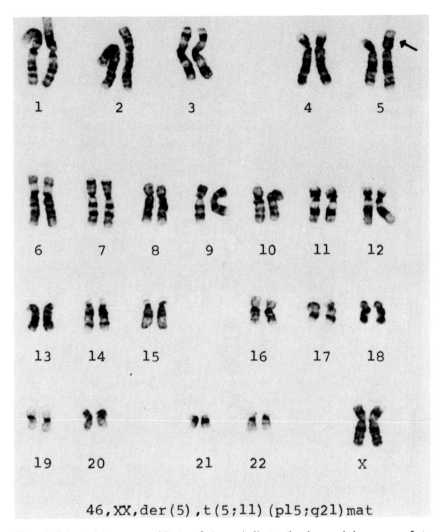

$$46,XX,der(5),t(5;11)(p15;q21)mat$$

Fig. 10. G-banded karyotype of *Patient 3.* Arrow indicates the abnormal chromosome 5p+.

is a certain overlap in clinical manifestations; eg microcephaly, micrognathia, and low-set ears may be found in both syndromes.

Table 1 presents a summary of the cytogenetic and prognostic data from the 13 cases. *Patients 4* and *5* were sibs, all others were presumably unrelated.

Five patients (*Nos. 8, 10, 11, 12,* and *13*) had 47 chromosomes including the 11q duplication—without associated deletion—and a partial duplication of

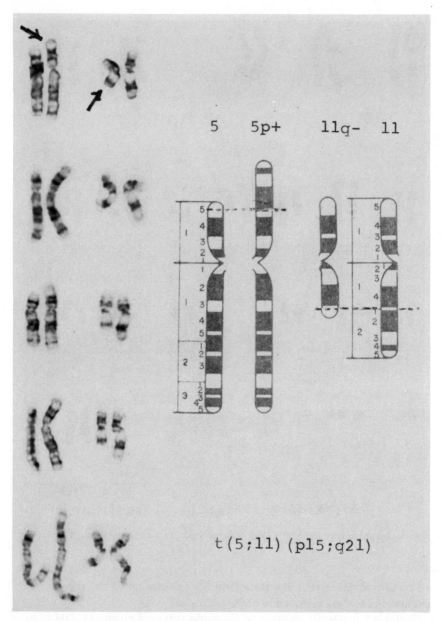

Fig. 11. Partial G-banded karyotypes from mother of *Patient 3*. Five sets of chromosome pairs 5 and 11, and an ideogram indicating the points of chromosome breakage and rejoining, demonstrate the truly reciprocal nature of this balanced translocation.

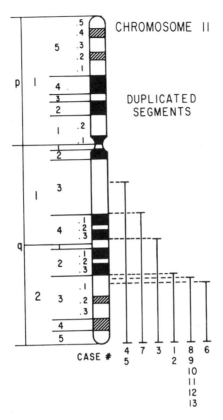

CHROMOSOME 11

DUPLICATED
SEGMENTS

CASE #

Fig. 12. Ideogram of chromosome 11 depicting G-bands and sub-bands as evident in early metaphases (modified from Paris Conference Standard Ideogram). The duplicated segments in 13 reported cases of 11q duplication are indicated by vertical bars. *Patients 1, 2,* and *3* are the subjects of this article. (References to *Patients 4* through *13* are given in Table 1.)

chromosome 22. An apparently identical reciprocal translocation t(11;22)(q23.1; q11.1) was found in one parent of each of these patients [6-9]. Because of the location of the breakpoints, this translocation can be expected to lead to unstable meiotic configurations. Nondisjunction involving the derivative chromosome 22, which consists of a 22 short arm and centromere with region 11q23.1→qter attached to it, gave rise to the "47, + small acrocentric" karyotypes found in the probands. The five families, all reported from France, were not known to be related. In two instances, the translocation was traced back over three and four generations respectively [7]; however, de novo occurrence of this t(11;22) translocation was not demonstrated in either kindred. Therefore, the number of original rearrangement events leading to apparently identical translocations cannot

TABLE 1. Duplication 11q Syndrome – Cytogenetic and Prognostic Data

Patient No.	Reference	Parental translocation	Sex	Age	Mental retardation
1	This article	t (6;11) (q27;q23.1) mat	M	1 yr	Severe
2	This article	t (4;11) (q35;q23.1) mat	F	∓ 5 wk	
3	This article	t (5;11) (p15;q21) mat	F	6 yr	Profound
4	Roth et al [3]	t (11;13) (q13;q32-34) pat	M	∓10 mo	+
5	ibid	same	F	∓ 1 wk	
6	Jacobsen et al [4]	t (11;21) (q23;q22) mat	M	11 yr	IQ 65
7	Tusques et al [5]	t (10;11) (q26;q13.3) pat	F	∓ 4 days	
8	Laurent et al [6]	t (11;22) (q23.1.911.1) mat	M	2 mo	+
9	ibid	t (11;17) (q23.1.;p13) mat	M	2 yr	IQ 50
10	Aurias et al [7]	t (11;22) (q23.1;q11.1) mat	M	1 mo	
11	ibid	t (11;22) (q23.1;q11.1) mat	F	∓ 1 hr	
12	Giraud et al [8]	t (11;22) (q23;q11) mat	F	∓ 1 day	
13	Ayraud et al [9]	t (11;22) (q23.1;q11.1) mat	M	4 yr	IQ <20

∓ = died

be determined. These reports should not be taken as evidence for the existence of preferred sites of breakage and exchange between chromosomes 11 and 22, although it is intriguing to speculate on possible homologous regions in different chromosomes. As has been recently demonstrated by Allderdice et al [10] in the case of a pericentric inversion of chromosome 3, apparently unrelated families carrying identical chromosomal rearrangements may have a distant common ancestor.

The most consistent clinical findings in the 13 liveborn patients with chromosomally proven dup(11)q syndrome are listed in Table 2 (Growth data) and in Table 3 (Anomalies). In addition, several kindreds contained one or more similarly affected members who were not karyotyped but are thought to have had the same syndrome.

The maternal uncle of *Patient 1* and the brother of *Patient 3* have been described in the respective case reports.

An older sister of *Patients 4* and *5* (*Case IV-23* in the original report [3]) had died at 16 days from cyanotic congenital heart disease. She had dysplastic clavicles and meningomyelocele. Three additional children of translocation carriers from the same kindred had died in infancy with malformations such as meningomyelocele, spina bifida, transposition of the great vessels, aplastic kidney, and biliary atresia. Other significant findings were uterus unicornis, inguinal hernia, and clubfeet.

TABLE 2. Duplication 11q Syndrome – Growth Data

Patient No.	Gestation (weeks)	Birthweight (gm)	Length (cm)	Postnatal growth delay
1	40	2300	48	+[b]
2	40	2600	49	nk
3	39	2250	nk[a]	+
4	38	1800	46	+
5	40	2380	48	nk
6	37	2250	50	+
7	42	2380	46	nk
8	42	2500	48	+
9	40	3040	49	–[c]
10	40	2330	46	nk
11	40	2350	48	nk
12	36	2350	47	nk
13	40	2380	48	+

[a] nk = not known.

[b] + present.

[c] – absent.

TABLE 3. Duplication 11q Syndrome – Anomalies

Anomalies	Patients with symptom present	Patients with available information
Microcephaly	. 8	10
Short nose/long philtrum	11	11
Microretrognathia	13	13
Retracted lower lip	10	12
Apparently low-set ears	9	12
Prominent anthelix	7	8
Palate–highly arched	4	10
Palate–cleft	6	13
Clavicular defect	3	3
Dysplastic acetabulum/ dislocated hip	4	5
Talipes equinovarus	4	6
Cardiac defect	11	11
Urinary tract malformation	5	8
Micropenis	6	7
Cutis laxa	6	9

Not included in Tables 2 and 3 was a 980 gm stillborn male, product of a 33-week gestation, who had craniorachischisis [11]. At autopsy, the pituitary gland was hypoplastic and lacked eosinophilic cells. The published karyotype, interpreted in terms of the Paris Nomenclature, would most likely be 46,XY,der(6), t(6;11) (p25;q23) pat, the abnormality consisting of duplication of region 11q23→qter and deletion of the 6p telomere.

The following summary of the dup(11)q syndrome is based on the 13 liveborn chromosomally proven cases listed in the tables as well as on the probably likewise affected relatives.

Growth deficiency of prenatal onset, moderate-to-profound mental retardation, and microcephaly were consistent manifestations. In the neonate, hypotonia of the trunk and hypertonia of the limbs, with abducted arms, flexed forearms, and clenched fists, were associated with feeding difficulties due to inability to suck or swallow [12].

The face is characterized by short nose, long philtrum, and small mandible with retracted lower lip. Hypotelorism was present in *Patient 1* and in his deceased maternal uncle. *Patients 4* and *5* had hypertelorism, while the interocular distances were apparently normal in the other patients. The external ears were large and often apparently low set or rotated backwards. They were characterized by poorly developed helices and prominent anthelices. Preauricular dimples or skin tags were common.

The palate was either cleft or high arched. Several patients presented with the complete Pierre-Robin anomaly consisting of microretrognathia, cleft posterior palate, and glossoptosis.

Congenital defects of cardiac development, most often a septal defect and/or patent ductus arteriosus, were found in the majority of cases. The impression of wide-spaced nipples was reported in three newborns with this syndrome (*Patients 8,9,10*). When internipple distances were measured in *Patients 1* and *3,* they were 20% and 22% of the chest circumferences, respectively, which was in the normal range for age.

Inguinal or umbilical hernias, urinary tract abnormalities, and developmental defects of female internal genitalia were occasionally present while common mesentery, aplastic hemidiaphragm, and hypoplastic gallbladder were reported in single cases only.

Some skeletal defects were frequently described such as dysplastic acetabulum with or without dislocated hip and talipes equinovarus; whereas kyphoscoliosis, radioulnar synostosis, and absent fibulas represented isolated findings. A developmental defect of one or both clavicles was demonstrated in four patients. *Patients 1* and *3* lacked fusion of the medial and the lateral portions of the right clavicle, and two sibs reported by Rott et al [3] had dysplastic clavicles similar to the findings in cleidocranial dysostosis. Shortened distal phalanges were reported in *Patients 3* and *13.*

Micropenis without hypospadias (Fig. 2) was present in seven of eight males. Normal response to testosterone, administered orally to *Patients 8* and *9* and locally in *Patient 1,* was documented by accelerated penile growth. *Patient 6* was reported to have had normal male genitalia at age 11. No information was given about the size of his penis at birth or of any previous hormone treatment.

Central nervous system malformations were variable. Neural tube closure defects, such as craniorachischisis and meningomyelocele, were reported once each. Agenesis of the corpus callosum was found in two autopsied cases, and decreased cellular elements in the pituitary gland were found in two others.

Lax, hyperextensible skin has been a frequent finding in the newborn period and was less prominent in older patients.

Dermatoglyphics included preponderance of whorls and ulnar loops on fingertips, interdigital patterns, and an increased distance between the palmar triradii a and b, due to radial displacement of a. This unusual characteristic has been documented in *Patients 1,3, 7,* and *10.*

The combination of retracted lower lip, clavicular defect, and micropenis appears unusual enough to allow clinical recognition of this syndrome at birth–at least in the male. Demonstration of the cytogenetic abnormality is necessary for diagnostic proof.

ACKNOWLEDGMENTS

The competent technical assistance of M.G. Brown, C. Kernahan, C. Bradshaw, and H. Müller is gratefully acknowledged.

We thank the consultant physicians K. Lyons Jones, W.F. Friedmann, D.H. Sutherland, T. Roth, M. Kaufhold, L.P. Newman, and J. Taylor, physical therapist, for contributing to the clinical evaluation of *Patient 1*.

REFERENCES

1. Francke U: Quinacrine mustard fluorescence of human chromosomes: Characterization of unusual translocations. Am J Hum Genet 24:189-213, 1972.
2. Mann J, Rafferty J: Cri-du-chat syndrome combined with partial C-group trisomy. J Med Genet 9:289-292, 1972.
3. Rott HD, Schwanitz G, Grosse KP, Alexandrow G: C11/D13-Translocation in four generations. Humangenetik 14:300-305, 1972.
4. Jacobsen P, Hauge M, Henningsen K, Hobolth N, Mikkelsen M, Philip J: An (11;21) translocation in four generations with chromosome 11 abnormalities in the offspring. Hum Hered 23:568-585, 1973.
5. Tusques J, Grislain JR, André M-J, Mainard R, Rival JM, Cadudal JL, Dutrillaux B, Lejeune J: Trisomie partielle 11q identifiée grace à l'étude en "dénaturation ménagée" par la chaleur, de la translocation équilibrée paternelle. Ann Genet (Paris) 15:167-172, 1972.
6. Laurent C, Biemont M-C, Bethenod M, Crêt L, David M: Deux observations de trisomie 11q (q23.1→qter) avec la même anomalie des organes génitaux externes. Ann Genet (Paris) 18:179-184, 1975.
7. Aurias A, Turc C, Michiels Y, Sinêt P-M, Graveleau D, Lejeune J: Deux cas de trisomie 11q (q23.1 → qter) par translocation t (11;22) (q23.1;q11.1) dans deux familles différentes. Ann Genet (Paris) 18:185-188, 1975.
8. Giraud F, Mattei J-F, Mattei M-G, Bernard R: Trisomie partielle 11q et translocation familial 11-22. Humangenetik 28:343-347, 1975.
9. Ayraud N, Galiana A, Llyod M, Deswarte M: Trisomie 11q (q23.1→qter) par translocation maternelle t (11;22) (q231; q11 1). Une nouvelle observation. Ann Genet (Paris) 19:65-68, 1976.
10. Allderdice PW, Browne N, Murphy DP: Chromosome 3 duplication q21 → qter deletion p25 → pter syndrome in children of carriers of a pericentric inversion inv(3) (p25q21). Am J Hum Genet 27:699-718, 1975.
11. Wright Y, Clark WE, Breg WR: Craniorachischisis in a partially trisomic 11 fetus in a family with reproductive failure and a reciprocal translocation, t (6p+;11q−). J Med Genet 11:69-75, 1974.
12. Aurias A, Laurent C: Trisomie 11q. Individualisation d'un nouveau syndrome. Ann Genet (Paris) 18:189-191, 1975.

A Case of Deletion of Short Arm of Chromosome 8

Jaakko Leisti, MD, and Pertti Aula, MD

We report a patient who has a de novo deletion of the short arm of chromosome 8, multiple anomalies, and developmental retardation.

CASE REPORT

The patient is a 6-month-old girl who was born one week before term to a 27-year-old mother and a 36-year-old father. The mother had two healthy children and no miscarriages. The family history was negative with respect to congenital anomalies or mental retardation.

The mother had recurrent headaches in early pregnancy and in the fifth month she had a seizure whose etiology could not be established. The remainder of the pregnancy, labor and delivery were normal. The baby received an Apgar rating of 9 at 1 and 5 min. The birthweight was 2,700 gm length 44 cm and head circumference 32 cm. The placenta appeared normal and weighed 460 gm.

Multiple anomalies were noticed soon after birth and a systolic heart murmur became audible at a few weeks of age. After recovering from mild RDS (respiratory distress syndrome), the baby continued having periods of cyanosis, respiratory difficulties, and feeding problems. She was digitalized at 2 months with partial improvement. Psychomotor development has been slow and her length and head circumference have increased slowly.

Examination at 3 months revealed a weight of 3,300 gm (4 SD below mean for age and sex), length of 52 cm (−4 SD) and head circumference of 35.5 cm (−4 SD). She needed a nasogastric tube for feeding, and developed dyspnea on exertion. Her head was narrow temporally and the occiput appeared prominent (Figs. 1

Birth Defects: Original Article Series, Volume XIII, Number 3B, pages 187−194

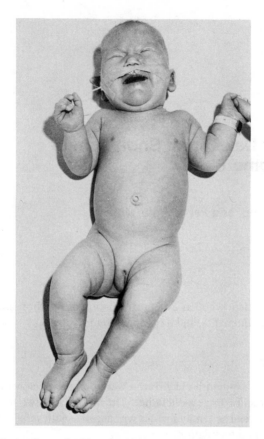

Fig. 1 The patient at 3 months. Note the widely spaced nipples and the puffiness of the hands and feet.

and 2). The sutures and fontanels were normal. The auricles were small and dysmorphic (Fig. 3). The palpebral fissures were narrow and widely spaced, with bilateral epicanthic folds. The eyes were small and there was a marked nystagmus. The nose was small and wide with a shallow bridge and anteverted nares. The mandible appeared protruding, and the mouth was small with down-turned corners. The palate was narrow anteriorly (Fig. 4). The neck was short with abundant skin at the nape. The nipples were wildly spaced. A III/VI systolic murmur was audible. The limbs were well proportioned and there was abundant subcutaneous tissue especially on hands and feet. The dermatoglyphic patterns appeared normal, and there was a transitional simian crease on the left palm. The toes were crowded with the 2nd and 4th overriding the others (Fig. 5).

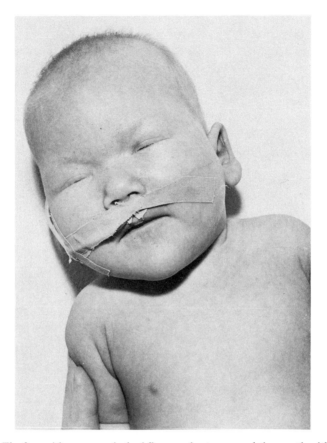

Fig. 2. The face with narrow palpebral fissures, short nose, and the mouth with down-turned corners.

Laboratory Findings

Pneumoencephalograms suggested mild central cerebral atrophy, without evidence of gross brain malformation. Skeletal roentgenograms were normal except for a hemivertebra at T8. Normal kidneys and collecting systems were seen in intravenous urograms. Tests for prenatally acquired infections, thyroid function, and amino acid excretion were normal. ECG and heart films were abormal and suggested a VSD (ventricular septal defect). The red cell glutathione reductase activity was about one-half of the normal activity, suggesting localization of the glutathione reductase gene in the deleted part of the short arm of chromosome 8 [1].

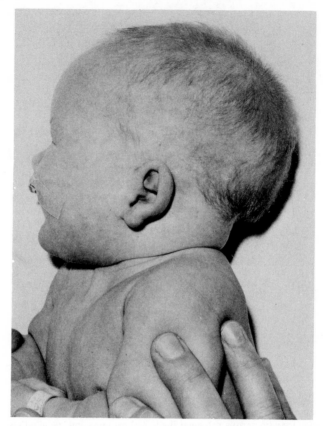

Fig. 3. Left profile. The occiput appears prominent, the chin protruding, and there is abundant skin around the nape. The pinnas are thick.

Cytogenetic Findings

Lymphocyte chromosomes were analyzed using both Giemsa and R-banding techniques. The chromosome number was 46. A deletion of the short arm of chromosome 8 was apparent in all analyzed cells while all other chromosomes were structurally normal (Fig. 6). The deletion involved most probably the distal portion of the short arm starting from the band "p21," although an interstitial deletion could not be ruled out. Thus the patient's karyotype was 46,XX,del(8) (:p21→qter). The parents' chromosomes were normal.

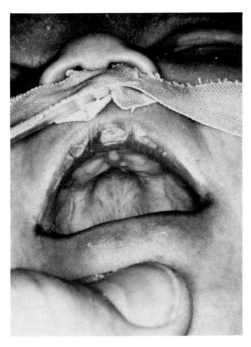

Fig. 4. The anteriorly narrow palate with prominent lateral ridges.

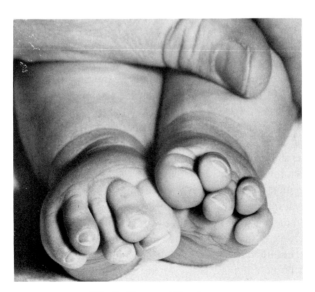

Fig. 5. The overriding toes.

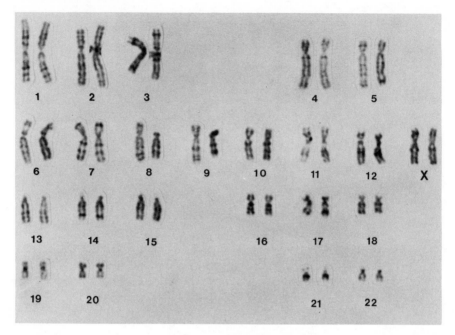

Fig. 6. Karyotype of the patient: 46,XX,del(8)(:p21→qter). Giemsa technique.

COMMENT

Deletions of autosomes are uncommon and are invariably associated with developmental abnormalities and retardation. Three additional 8p— cases were found in the literature, and their clinical data are presented in Table 1. The deletion in the case of Lubs and Lubs [2] was due to a maternal balanced translocation, while the deletions in the cases of Taillemite et al [3] and Orye and Craen [4] were sporadic and resembled the one in our patient.

Comparison of the four cases and their combined data (Table 2) indicates that deletion of the short arm of chromosome 8 has a disturbing effect on fetal and postnatal development. All patients were retarded and three suffered also from poor growth. Congenital heart defect was present in three patients. A variety of other dysmorphic features was present, and it is possible that the deletion gives rise to a specific dysmorphogenic syndrome, although only two of the four cases seemed to have similarities in their patterns of somatic anomalies (present case and Orye and Craen). These included narrow forehead, midfacial abnormalities, and the peculiarly dysmorphic pinnas. However, at this point the clinical variability is too great and the number of known cases too small for a definite delineation of a new syndrome.

TABLE 1. Clinical Features of 8p− Patients

	Present case	Lubs and Lubs (1973)	Taillemite et al (1975)	Orye and Craen (1976)
Sex	Female	Female	Male	Male
Age	3 months	4 years, 8 months	13 years	4 months; 6 years, 10 months
Birthweight	2,700 gm	2,380 gm	2,200 gm	3,700 gm
Height	−4 SD	−2 SD	Normal	Normal; − 2 SD
Head circumference	−4 SD	−1 SD	Normal	Normal
Cranium	Narrow temporally, prominent occiput	Normal	Shallow forehead	Narrow
Eyes	Epicanthic folds, telecanthus	Epicanthic folds	Epicanthic fold	Epicanthic folds
Nose	Small and broad, flat nasal bridge		Long	Flat nasal bridge
Mouth	Small, down-turned corners	Wide and thin, cleft palate	Normal	Malaligned teeth
Chin	Wide, protruding tip			Retrognathy
Auricles	Small, dysmorphic	Normal	Normal	Low-set, abnormal consistency
Neck	Short, abundant skin	Short, thick	Normal	Short
Chest	Wide-set nipples	Wide-set nipples, depressed sternum	Wide-set nipples, depressed sternum	Broad, wide-set nipples
Heart	Congenital heart defect (?VSD)	Systolic murmur	VSD, PS	Normal
Genitalia	Normal	Normal	Testicular hypoplasia	Normal
Upper limbs	Puffy hands, left simian crease	Normal	Left simian crease	Puffy hands, t″ triradius
Lower limbs	Puffy feet, overriding toes	Normal	Normal	Parapatellar dimples
Development	Retarded psychomotor, slow growth	Moderately retarded, slow growth	Grossly retarded	Retarded, slow growth
Other findings	Mild central cerebral atrophy, hemivertebra			Recurrent nephrolithiasis

TABLE 2. Most Significant Features in the Four 8p— Cases

	Anomaly	Frequency
Developmental	Developmental retardation	4/4
	Intrauterine growth retardation	3/4
	Postnatal growth retardation	3/4
Craniofacial	Narrow forehead	2/4
	Shallow bridge of nose	2/4
	Epicanthic folds	4/4
	Dysmorphic auricles	2/4
	Dysmorphic mandible	2/4
Limbs	Puffy hands and feet	2/4
	Simian crease	2/4
Cardiovascular	Congenital heart defect	3/4
Other	Wide-set nipples	3/4
	Depressed sternum	2/4
	Hypoplastic testes	1/2

ACKNOWLEDGMENTS

This work was supported by the Foundation for Pediatric Research in Finland.

REFERENCES

1. de la Chapelle A, Icén A, Aula P, Leisti J, Turleau C, de Grouchy J: Mapping of the gene for glutathione reductase on chromosome 8. Ann Génét (Paris) 19:253–256, 1976.
2. Lubs HA, Lubs ML: New cytogenetic technics applied to a series of children with mental retardation. In Caspersson T, Zech L (eds): "Chromosome Identification — Technique and Applications in Biology and Medicine." Nobel Symposia 23. New York: Academic Press, 1973, pp 241–250.
3. Taillemite J-L, Channarond J, Tinel H, Mulliez N, Roux C: Délétion partielle du bras court du chromosome 8. Ann Génét (Paris) 18:21.
4. Orye E, Craen M: A new chromosome deletion syndrome. Report of a patient with a 46,XY,8p— chromosome constitution. Clin Genet 9:289–301, 1976.

Familial Gingival Fibromatosis Associated With Progressive Deafness in Five Generations of a Family

Gilbert Jones, MD, Robert S. Wilroy, Jr, MD, and Verna McHaney, MCD

Gingival hyperplasia is a slowly progressive enlargement of gingival tissue often associated with other phenotypic abnormalities and is frequently inherited in an autosomal dominant or autosomal recessive manner. The gingivae are normal in color, stippled, nonpainful, and do not bleed readily [1–3]. They may be either nodular or smooth on inspection [4]. The normal eruption of the permanent teeth appears to be the stimulus for gingival enlargement, although enlargement may occur at eruption of the deciduous teeth, or may be congenital [5, 6].

The Genetics Section of the Department of Pediatrics of the University of Tennessee Center for the Health Sciences has recently investigated the family of an 11-year-old white male referred to us by the University of Tennessee College of Dentistry.

CASE REPORT

The family history (Fig. 1) reveals that individuals with gingival hyperplasia have appeared in five generations. Many maternal relatives have also manifested hearing loss that becomes symptomatic late in the second decade of life. In our investigation of this family, eight individuals have been evaluated clinically and audiometrically by the authors (Fig. 1). Historical data are available on an additional 40 persons.

The proband's psychomotor development was normal (*V-15* in Fig. 1). He entered school at 5 years and is currently in the 6th grade. He has never taken diphenylhydantoin. Acute ear trauma, prolonged exposure to loud or high-pitched noises, and the use of ototoxic drugs are denied.

Birth Defects: Original Article Series, Volume XIII, Number 3B, pages 195–201
© 1977 The National Foundation

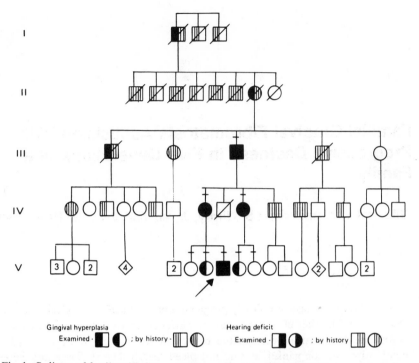

Fig. 1. Pedigree of family with five generations affected with gingival fibromatosis and progressive deafness. A horizontal line above a symbol denotes evaluation by the authors.

The boy weighed 23 kg and was 128 cm tall. The skull was normal. The patient was not hirsute. The intercanthal distance was 3.2 cm. Facial features were otherwise unremarkable (Fig. 2). The pupils and fundi were normal. The pinnae were large and protruded from the skull. The external auditory canals and tympanic membranes were normal, as was the nose. The alveolar ridges were broad. Twelve upper and 12 lower teeth had erupted. Of these, four upper and four lower teeth were permanent. The premaxilla was prominent. The patient had obvious gingival hyperplasia, most prominent anteriorly with gingival tissue extending well over the teeth. The remainder of the physical findings were within normal limits.

Histologic examination (Fig. 3) of the gingivae revealed edema and moderate vascularity of the lamina propria, thickening of the superficial epithelium, and increased size of the rete pegs. Areas of increased fibroblasts were apparent. Epithelial metaplasia to keratin formation, which may have been caused by repeated trauma, was evident. Whorls of mature collagen were mixed with nests of immature collagen, implying that active production of collagen was still occurring.

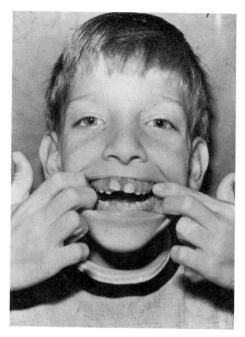

Fig. 2. Proband, *V-15*, illustrating gingival hyperplasia and a prominent premaxilla.

Results of CBC, serum electrolytes, urinalysis, and metabolic screen were normal. Serum thyroxine levels were normal. VDRL was negative. Chromosome analysis revealed an apparently normal 46,XY karyotype. Dental x rays revealed disorientation of the unerupted permanent teeth, and deviation of the teeth from a normal right angle with the surrounding bone.

Audiometry revealed significant bilateral symmetric hearing loss above 2,000 Hz with normal function below that frequency. Impedence audiometry revealed, at 4,000 Hz, a reduced sensation level to produce the stapedial reflex threshold. This was consistent with the recruitment phenomenon present in cochlear hearing loss.

The proband's 43-year-old mother (Fig. 4) experienced a progressive hearing loss late in the second decade of life and now she must read lips. Except for the presence of hyperplastic gingivae, findings on physical examination were normal. Her gingivae were hypertrophied, predominantly in the anterior part of the mouth, and were pink, stippled, and nodular. The premaxilla was prominent. Audiometric examination revealed loss of hearing to 60 db at 6,000 Hz and loss to 45 db in the lower frequencies.

The proband's maternal grandfather, age 60, had gingival hyperplasia that had

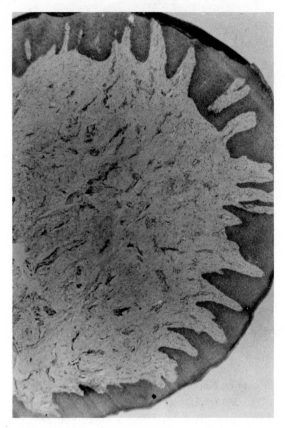

Fig. 3. Histologic features of proband's gingiva, illustrating edema of lamina propria, thickened superficial epithelium, and increased size of rete pegs.

been treated by complete dental extraction and gingivectomy. He related that he had worked in a machine shop with constant loud noise exposure for the past 20 years. However, he was clinically "hard of hearing" before beginning to work there. Physical examination revealed normal findings except for the presence of false teeth. His audiogram revealed hearing loss of 60 db at frequencies above 1,500 Hz, with loss to 30 db below that frequency.

The proband's 20-year-old sister also had gingival hyperplasia with a prominent premaxilla. Audiometric testing revealed no significant functional loss. A 21-year-old sister had neither gingival hyperplasia nor significant hearing loss.

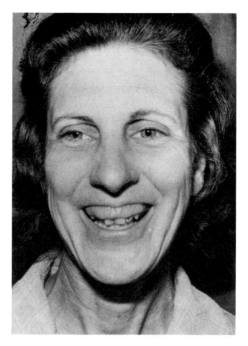

Fig. 4. Mother of proband, *IV-8,* with gingival hyperplasia.

The proband's maternal aunt, who was 38 years old, related having had hyperplasia of her gingivae treated by gingivectomy and extraction of her maxillary and mandibular incisors, which have been replaced by prostheses. Audiometry revealed symmetric hearing loss of 30–40 db below 1,500 Hz. Her older daughter (*V-16* in Fig. 1), had gingival hyperplasia but no hearing deficit while her 20-year-old daughter (*V-17* in Fig. 1), had neither gingival hyperplasia nor significant hearing loss by audiogram.

By history, an additional 28 individuals were said to have gingival hyperplasia. Of these, 15 demonstrated symptomatic hearing loss. *No individual complained of hearing loss who did not also manifest gingival hyperplasia.*

The pedigree (Fig. 1) shows that gingival hyperplasia has occurred in five generations, the individual first known to be affected being the proband's great-great grandfather. Family photographs confirmed the presence of gingival hyperplasia in *I–1* and *II–7*. Gingival hyperplasia appears to be transmitted in an autosomal dominant fashion in this family.

DISCUSSION

Gingival hyperplasia as an isolated phenomenon can be inherited in either an autosomal dominant or autosomal recessive manner [4, 6–9]. It has also been reported in association with several other abnormalities, the most common being hypertrichosis. Frequently such individuals have been mentally retarded, and both autosomal dominant and autosomal recessive inheritance has been proposed [10–13].

Gingival hyperplasia in association with multiple soft tissue, nail, and cartilage defects, skeletal and joint abnormalities, and visceromegaly, has been reported as an autosomal dominantly inherited abnormality [2, 14]. A family has been described in which gingival hyperplasia and multiple hyaline fibromata have apparently been inherited in an autosomal recessive manner [1]. Sporadic cases of gingival hyperplasia in association with virginal breast hypertrophy, hypertrichosis, mental retardation, and skeletal abnormalities have been described [1]. A syndrome involving gingival hyperplasia, hypopigmentation, microphthalmia, mental retardation, spasticity and athetoid movements has been reported and probably is inherited as an autosomal recessive condition [1]. The triad of gingival hyperplasia, failure of eruption of teeth, and corneal dystrophy has been transmitted as an autosomal dominant disorder [15, 16]. Gingival hyperplasia has also been described in patients with mucolipidosis type II [17]. Hearing loss that becomes symptomatic late in the second decade of life has apparently not previously been reported in association with gingival hyperplasia.

SUMMARY

Gingival hyperplasia may be inherited in a variety of ways, usually in an autosomal dominant or autosomal recessive manner. Additional phenotypic abnormalities are frequently associated with the gingival hyperplasia. To our knowledge, the family described here represents the first instance of autosomal dominantly inherited gingival hyperplasia associated with progressive neural hearing loss.

ACKNOWLEDGMENTS

This work was supported in part by Special Project No. 900, Division of Health Services, MCHS, HSMHA, DHEW, and a grant from the National Foundation—March of Dimes.

REFERENCES

1. Witkop CJ: Heterogeneity in gingival fibromatosis. In Bergsma D (ed): Part XI. "Orofacial Structures." Baltimore: Williams & Wilkins for The National Foundation— March of Dimes, BD: OAS VII (7):210, 1971.
2. Alavandar G: Elephantiasis gingivae, J All-India Dent Assoc 37:349, 1965.
3. Hine MK: Fibrous hyperplasia of gingivae. J Am Dent Assoc 44:681, 1952.
4. Zegarelli EV, Kutscher AH, Lichtenthal R: Idiopathic gingival hyperplasia: Report of 20 cases. Am J Dig Dis 8:782, 1963.
5. Henefer EP: Congenital idiopathic gingival hyperplasia with deciduous dentition. Oral Surg 24:65, 1967.
6. Ruggles SD: Primary hypertrophy of the gums. JAMA 84:20, 1925.
7. Rapp R, Nikiforuk G, Donohue DW, Williams CHM: Idiopathic hyperplasia of gingivae associated with macrocheilia and ankyloglossia: A case report. J Periodontol 26:51, 1955.
8. Becker W, Collings CK, Zimmerman ER, De La Rosa M, Singdalsen D: Hereditary gingival fibromatosis. Oral Surg 24:313, 1967.
9. Garn SM, Hatch CE: Hereditary general gingival hyperplasia. J Hered 41:41, 1950.
10. Byars LT, Sarnat BG: Congenital macrogingivae (fibromatosis gingivae) and hypertrichosis. Surgery 15:964, 1944.
11. Zackin SJ, Weisberger D: Hereditary gingival fibromatosis: Report of a family. Oral Surg 14:828, 1961.
12. Perkoff D: Primary generalized hypertrophy of the gums. Dent Rec 49:411, 1929.
13. Winter GB, Simkiss MJ: Hypertrichosis with hereditary gingival hyperplasia. Arch Dis Child 49:394, 1974.
14. Laband PF, Habib G, Humphreys GS: Hereditary gingival fibromatosis. Oral Surg 17:339, 1964.
15. Rutherfurd ME: Three generations of inherited dental defect. Br Med J 2:9, 1931.
16. Houston IB, Shotts N: Rutherfurd's syndrome. A familial oculodental disorder. Acta Paediatr (Uppsala) 55:233, 1966.
17. Reed WD, Sugarman G: Inclusion cell disease. Arch Dermatol 106:411, 1972.

CASE REPORTS

A — SYNDROME OF MENTAL RETARDATION, CLEFT PALATE, EVENTRATION OF DIAPHRAGM, CONGENITAL HEART DEFECT, GLAUCOMA, GROWTH FAILURE AND CRANIOSYNOSTOSIS

A female patient was born after 38½ weeks gestation by vertex presentation and normal delivery. Birthweight was 2,450 gm, length 48 cm, and head circumference 30.5 cm. On intrauterine growth charts the length was just below the 50th percentile, weight just above the 10th percentile, and head circumference below the 10th percentile. The mother received an antibiotic at approximately 5 months' gestation, but the pregnancy was otherwise normal until term when slight bleeding occurred. The parents were 29 years old, of German origin but unrelated. The mother had two previous spontaneous miscarriages at 8 weeks gestation followed by the birth of a normal son in 1970. The family history revealed no other instances of birth defects in any way similar to the proband.

At birth she was noted to have proptosis, a prominent beaked nose, mild downward slanting palpebral fissures, abnormal ears (particularly the right) (Figs. 1 and 2), and an incomplete cleft of the secondary palate (Fig. 3). There was a palpable mass at the lateral edge of the left supraorbital ridge which was presumed to be a dermoid cyst. The nails were narrow and hyperconvex, especially on the 4th and 5th fingers. She developed cyanotic spells, and subsequent investigation revealed eventration of the left diaphragm and a congenital heart defect which required treatment with Digoxin for mild congestive failure. The fontanels and sutures were open. She was unable to close her eyelids completely; however, there was no clouding of the corneas and the corneal diameters were 9 mm (normal). Brushfield spots were present and the optic nerve heads showed moderately prominent cups.

Birth Defects: Original Article Series, Volume XIII, Number 3B, pages 203—228
© 1977 **The National Foundation**

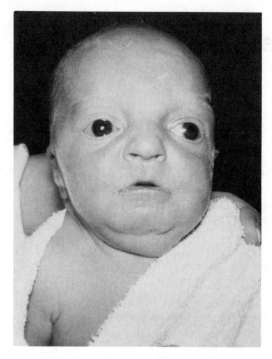

Fig. 1. The patient at age 1 week showing proptosis, divergent squint, and mild downward slanting palpebral fissures.

Special investigations at this time revealed a normal urine amino acid screening and chromatography. T4 was 11.8 μg% and a leukocyte culture revealed an apparently normal female karyotype (46,XX). Roentgenograms disclosed the following: chest — there was a considerable portion of large and possibly small bowel in the left lower hemithorax with displacement of the heart and mediastinum to the right: skull — apart from the vault being smaller than normal, the contour was normal as was the thickness and mineralization. Fontanels and sutures were normal and no calcification was seen; cervical spine — normal in AP, lateral, and oblique projections; optic foramina — normal; skeletal maturation corresponded to 38 weeks' gestation. An EEG was abnormal, with asymmetry and evidence of moderate disturbance of cerebral function maximal in the right hemisphere but with a diffuse disturbance throughout. Standard hemogram and urinalysis were normal. Serum electrolytes, glucose, calcium, phosphate, and alkaline phosphatase were normal. Blood urea nitrogen (BUN) was normal.

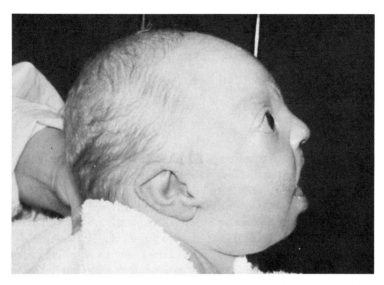

Fig. 2. Note proptosis, prominent nose, posterior slant, abnormal helix, and low-set ear with preauricular fistula. Age 1 week.

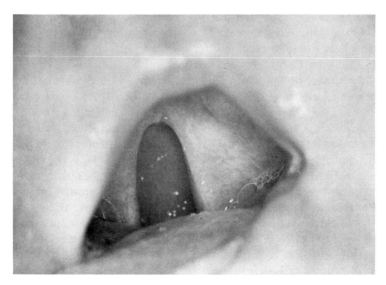

Fig. 3. U-Shaped incomplete cleft of secondary palate.

Dermatoglyphics

These showed a preponderance of nondiagnostic ulnar loops, the ridges were poorly developed in places with stippled patterns.

	1	2	3	4	5	Tri	Simian	Hallucal
R	Lu	Lu	Lu	Lu	Lu	t^1	—	Ld
L	Lu	W	Lu	W	Lu	t	—	Ld

Further Progress

At 4 months, gastric obstruction occurred, and she required surgery for gastric volvulus and the left diaphragmatic hernia. At this time it was noted that she was paying very little attention to her environment and that her development was slow. Her growth remained slow with a weight of 3.1 kg, length of 49.5 cm, and head circumference of 35 cm (all below the 3rd percentile). The fontanels and sutures remained open and there was no clinical evidence of glaucoma. A repeat leukocyte culture with Giemsa banding of the chromosomes was normal. At 9 months cardiac catheterization revealed a left to right shunt with an atrial septal defect, pulmonary stenosis, and a possible ventricular septal defect. Examination of her eyes under anesthesia revealed intraocular pressures of 13 and 14 mm Hg in the left and right eyes, respectively. The corneal diameters of 12.5 and 12 mm were slightly larger than normal but the pressures were well within normal limits. Development and growth continued to be slow.

At 10 months she developed seizures. The first one was mainly left-sided but very prolonged, lasting approximately 6 hours and leaving her with a residual left hemiparesis. Investigation of seizures disclosed normal serum calcium, phosphate, glucose, electrolytes, and cerebrospinal fluid. An EEG showed marked disturbance of function in the right hemisphere which was maximal in the parietotemporal area. Skull roentgenograms showed that the facial bones were small as compared to the vault, which itself was small, and that there was no suture closure. A brain scan with technetium[99] was normal and a bilateral carotid angiogram showed slightly enlarged ventricles bilaterally but was otherwise unremarkable. Because her proptosis seemed to be getting worse and there was evidence of left optic atrophy, right and left craniotomies with decompression of the orbits were carried out at 1 year of age. The previously mentioned supraorbital mass was removed and found to be a dermoid cyst. At this time she was noted to have bilateral inferior corneal erosions. The left optic nervehead had improved in color postoperatively. At 19 months, the EEG showed depression of activity in the right hemisphere; however, there were also some abnormalities noted in the left hemisphere. She underwent repair of her cleft palate, and her eyes were examined under anesthesia with no evidence of glaucoma; however left optic atrophy was again noted.

Since the left eye began to enlarge, she was again examined under anesthesia at 22 months and left-sided glaucoma was noted. The left cornea was slightly grey in appearance and there was increased photophobia. The intraocular pressure in the right eye was 8 mm Hg and in the left 32 mm Hg. Corneal diameters remained at 12 (right) and 13 cm. A left goniotomy was performed. She received phenobarbital and later diphenylhydantoin for her seizures.

Examination at 2 years 1 month revealed psychomotor retardation. Her length of 76 cm, weight of 7 kg, and head circumference of 41.9 cm were all abnormally small and well below the 3rd percentile. Her face suggested Crouzon syndromes (Figs. 4 and 5). Dental development was delayed with only two fully erupted (lower incisors) and two partially erupted teeth (upper molars). Her liver and spleen were not palpable and the external genitalia were normal. The previously mentioned left hemiparesis including left facial palsy was evident.

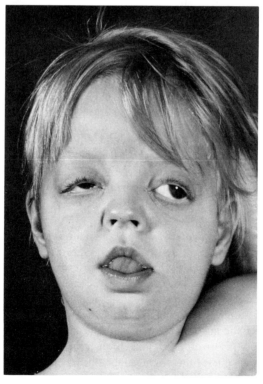

Fig. 4. At 2 years. Note prominent tongue, open mouth, short upper lip. The eyelids are unable to completely cover the eyes.

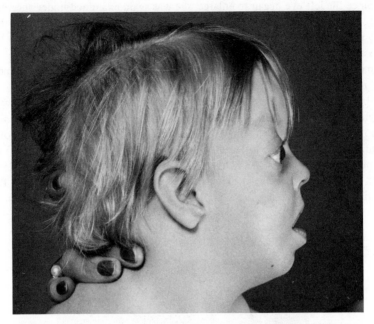

Fig. 5. At 2 years. Ears show evidence of postnatal development with improvement in shape of helix; prominent eyes and protruding lower lip are evident.

She was unable to sit or roll over but could hold her head up. There were considerable feeding difficulties. She developed pneumonia and this, coupled with further seizures and hyponatremia suggestive of inappropriate antidiuretic hormone production, finally resulted in her death at 29 months of age.

Postmortem

The anterior fontanel measured 1.5 X 1.3 cm; however, no visible sutures were seen in the skull except the frontoparietal sutures. The right cerebral hemisphere was smaller than the left. Sectioning revealed that the right frontal horn was larger than the left; however, the right caudate nucleus and probably the thalamus and lenticular nucleus were all smaller than those on the left side. The corpus callosum was very thin, measuring no more than 2 mm at any point. The cortex and white matter were unremarkable and showed no suggestion of previous infarction. Horizontal sections through the brainstem and cerebellum showed relative smallness of the right cerebral peduncle, right side of the pons, and possibly the right medullary pyramid. The cerebellar hemispheres and white matter were unremarkable as was the spinal cord. Microscopic sections showed a diffuse ischemic encephalopathy involving both cerebral cortex and basal ganglia. There was atrophy and gliosis of the left cortex, putamen, anterior rim of interior capsule, and thalamus consistent with old focal ischemic damage. The sections also showed focal cerebellar sclerosis bilaterally and confirmed the hypoplasia of the corpus callosum. The eyes both showed identical measurements as follows: AP diameter 20 mm, horizontal 19 mm, vertical 19 mm, cornea 12 mm horizontally and vertically 11 mm. Microscopic sections were unremarkable. In the cardiovascular system there was both right atrial and right ventricular hypertrophy. There was a large atrial septal defect measuring 12 mm in diameter, and the coronary sinus was smaller than normal. The pulmonary valve was bicuspid and measured 3 cm in circumference, however, there was no anatomic pulmonary obstruction. The ductus arteriosus was closed and there was no ventricular septal defect. The lungs were congested and microscopic sections showed a severe purulent bronchopneumonia. The remaining organs were present and normal.

COMMENT

The initial impression on seeing this child was one of the Crouzon syndome; however, it is apparent that she had a congenital cerebral defect plus malformations in several areas, and we believe that she represents an example of a true multiple congenital anomaly-mental retardation syndrome (MCA-MR) rather. than Crouzon syndrome. Mental deficiency has been observed in some cases of Crouzon syndrome as has epilepsy, glaucoma, and oligodontia, but to our knowledge no patient with Crouzon syndrome has had this severe degree of congenital microcephaly. The skull sutures remained open until at least 10 months of age as evidenced by the roentgenograms; however, these were unfortunately not repeated and craniosynostosis did take place within the next year since it was found at postmortem. Although the Crouzon syndrome is characterized by variable expressivity, this cannot be invoked in the present case since the parental skulls and facies show no evidence whatsoever of the syndrome. Christian et al [1] reported the combination of craniosynostosis with microcephaly, cleft palate, and arthrogryposis. Many of the features were secondary to abnormal neurologic development, and perhaps should not be considered as a true arthrogryposis. Our patient may belong in the same category. We suggest that the sutural closing was a passive event due to the underlying microencephaly and not a true active premature craniosynostosis as in the syndromes reviewed by Cohen [2].

SUMMARY

A patient is reported with a syndrome of mental retardation, congenital microcephaly, cleft palate, congenital heart defect, eventration of the diaphragm, optic atrophy, and glaucoma. Her facies was Crouzon-like, and cranio-synostosis, although not present at 10 months, was demonstrated postmortem at 29 months. It is suggested that she is an example of a true multiple congenital anomaly-mental retardation syndrome rather than an example of Crouzon syndrome with additional anomalies.

ACKNOWLEDGMENTS

The authors would like to acknowledge the help of many of their faculty colleagues and resident staff who were involved with the care of this patient. This work was supported in part by Medical Research Council of Canada grant No. MA 4539.

REFERENCES

1. Christian JC, Andrews PA, Conneally PM, Muller J: Autosomal recessive disease with arthrogryposis, dysmyelination, craniostenosis, and cleft palate. Clin Gent 2:95, 1971.
2. Cohen MM: An etiologic and nosologic overview of craniosynostosis syndromes. In Bergsma D (ed): "Malformation Syndromes." Excerpta Medica for The National Foundation—March of Dimes. BD:OAS XI(2):137–189, 1975.

R. B. Lowry
J. R. MacLean

B — SYNDROME OF MYOPATHY, SHORT STATURE, SEIZURES, RETINITIS PIGMENTOSA, AND CLEFT LIP

The patient was born in 1969, the third child to normal, healthy, unrelated white parents. The pregnancy, labor, and delivery were uncomplicated, and his birth-weight at term was 3,884 gm. His older sister and brother are 12 and 10 years old respectively and are normal. He sat at 7 months but did not crawl or explore much. He walked at 15 months and used single words up to the age of 4 years, but his receptive language developed normally. Toilet training was complete at 3 years and he was dry at night.

At 5 years of age he was referred for investigation of delayed growth and de-velopment. Psychologic testing indicated that he functioned at the 3 year, 9 month level (chronologic age 5 years, 4 months) with little scatter on test re-sults. His hearing appeared normal. At 6 years, 1 month, growth hormone assays by means of arginine and insulin infusions were performed and the results were within normal limits. At that time he was noted to be tired and to have droopy eyelids. An electromyogram (EMG) was suggestive of a myopathy.

The family history revealed that the father has a male first cousin with profound retardation and hypotonia, generalized muscle weakness, bilateral cleft lip and cleft palate, short stature (less than third percentile), nystagmus, severe bilateral clubfeet, wasting of thenar and hypothenar muscles, and bilateral inguinal herniae. Results of banded chromosome studies on this boy were normal as was his urinary amino acid chromatography. He is in one of the Provincial residential schools for the mentally retarded and was examined there by the authors. While he has some features in common with the propositus, nevertheless his total picture appears quite different.

Examination of the proband at 6 years, 10 months, revealed a quiet, cooperative child with obvious short stature, muscle weakness, and a tendency to frown or wrinkle his forehead when looking at people or objects. Height was 95.5

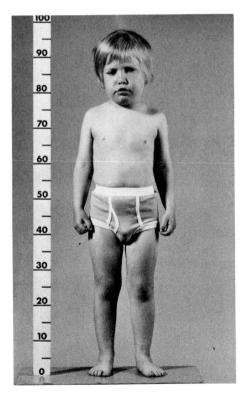

Fig. 1. Patient at age 6 years, 10 months. Note normal-looking muscle mass and general phenotype.

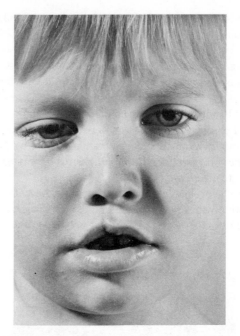

Fig. 2. Drooping of both lids is noted but more marked on right. Note incomplete cleft of the lip on right side.

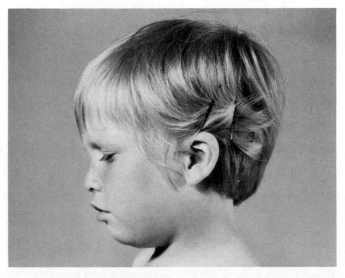

Fig. 3. Profile of patient showing small ear with thickened helix.

cm, weight 14 kg (both less than third percentile), lower segment 42.5 cm, and upper segment/lower segment ratio 1.25. Inner canthal distance was 2.9 cm, inter-pupillary 5.4 cm, and outer canthal 8.4 cm (all between 50th and 75th per-centile). Total hand length (right) was 10.8 cm (palm length 6.3 cm). There was ptosis of eyelids, more marked on right (Figs. 1 and 2) and an incomplete right cleft lip consisting of a small notch in the vermilion border but not extending into the alveolus. The pupils were normal and eye movements full; however, fundi showed diffuse pigmentation of retina. The palate was intact and there was no evidence of a submucous cleft palate. He had a full primary dentition, apart from normal loss of both lower central incisors. Both ears were small (Fig. 3), with thickening of the helix, length of left ear 5 cm, of right ear 4.5 cm (both approxi-mately third percentile). Hands, digits, and nails were normal. Feet showed bi-lateral clinodactyly of 5th toes but nails were normal. Heart and lungs were nor-mal. Liver size was normal (1 cm); spleen and kidneys were not palpable. He had a normal male genitalia with both testes descended. Muscle tone and power were decreased. When lying supine he could not get up unless he rolled over and "climbed upon himself" (Gowers sign). The deep tendon reflexes were normal and there were no Babinski reflexes. Sensation was normal. Cranial nerves were normal except for weakness of the sternocleidomastoids. There was no ataxia and the finger-nose test was performed well.

Investigations

Standard hemogram and urinalysis were normal, urine amino acid screening with ferric chloride, Benedict, nitroprusside, and MPS negative, and urine amino acid chromatogram normal. Serum sodium potassium, chloride, bicarbonate, calcium, and phosphate were normal. Alkaline phosphatase was normal. Serum creatine phosphokinase was normal (51 IU, range 17–110), and serum lactic de-hydrogenase (LDH) elevated (461 IU, normal range 50–150 IU/liter). The T4, effective thyroxin ratio (ETR), serum cholesterol, and triglyceride were normal. Beta lipoproteins were increased. Cerebrospinal fluid was normal. Chromosome karyotype from a Giemsa banded preparation was apparently normal (46,XY).

Roentgenographic Studies

Skull was normal and skeletal age approximately 3 years, which was more than 2 SD below the mean for his chronologic age of 6 years, 5 months. Skeletal survey showed slight generalized demineralization but no abnormal tubulation or unusual densities. The muscle mass in the upper arm appeared less than ex-pected. Chest was normal.

Electrodiagnostic Studies

Electroencephalogram (EEG) showed no focal, lateralizing activity, or frank epileptiform activity and was considered within normal limits for the age. Visual evoked potential (VER) and electroretinogram (ERG) recordings: VER potentials were of normal configuration over both left and right hemisphere and in the midline. Latency to the first major negative peak was approximately 80 msec, which was within normal range for his age. The ERG was very low in amplitude and indicated markedly abnormal function in the retinal cells with marked prolongation in latency. Electromyogram (EMG) was suggestive of a myopathy. Nerve conduction velocity (NCV) and electrocardiogram (ECG) were normal. Tests for myasthenia gravis using increasing evoked action potentials showed a normal endplate conduction.

Dermatoglyphics

	1	2	3	4	5	<atd.	Hallucal pattern
R	W	Lr	Lu	W	W	54°	Loop distal
L	Lu	W	Lu	W	W	53°	Arch fibular

Muscle Studies

A muscle biopsy was obtained from the vastus lateralis and it showed normal skeletal muscle by standard histologic techniques. Electron microscopy showed no abnormality of myofibrils, nor of the tubular system or mitochrondria. Many glycogen granules were present and the sarcolemmal nuclei were unremarkable. A striking feature was the presence of multiple concentric laminated bodies that were subsarcolemmal in location. Glycogen granules were present in the center of some of these laminated bodies, which occasionally appear in longitudinal section and are cylindrical.

FURTHER PROGRESS

In recent months the patient has developed seizures. During the first of these, which occurred while he was asleep in a car, both arms and legs began to jerk simultaneously. There was no incontinence nor tongue biting and the episode lasted about 0.5 min. Afterwards he was wide awake. Five more such episodes have occurred and he has been placed on Meberal 30 mg t.i.d. The mother also noted that he had developed spells after he had voided urine. These consisted of his arms dropping by his sides, fists clenched, and a grinning expression and backward rolling of his head. These last about 10 sec and have occurred 3–4 times a day but occasionally not at all. A cystoscopy was done, which was normal, as was a repeat urinalysis. Reexamination disclosed no new physical signs. Muscle enzyme studies again showed elevation of LDH and normal CPK. LDH isoenzymes were normal. Serum calcium was again normal (10.3 mg%) and serum lactate was mildly elevated (3.6 mmole/1; range 0.7–2.0). Blood gases and pH were normal. Blood amino acids showed a normal pattern. Serum hexosaminidase showed 560 nmoles/hr/ml of serum (95% range 400–900) with percentage A 57% (95% range 52.5–68.5%). Leukocyte enzymes hexosaminidase, beta galactosidase, and arylsulfatase A were normal. EEG showed no specific diagnostic features but was abnormal. VER had changed significantly from the previous test and was very abnormal at all three occipital locations. This suggested deterioration in function of the visual pathways through the hemispheres. Although the ERG had changed and appeared more normal than previously, it was still abnormal, indicating persistent evidence of disturbed retinal function. Computerized tomography (CT) scan showed no abnormality. ECG showed low voltages, possibly within normal limits but consistent with a myopathy. Audiometry showed a very mild air bone gap with mild conductive hearing loss but thresholds were probably elevated due to the child's inattention and the result is not considered significant.

SUMMARY

A five-year-old boy is presented with an undifferentiated myopathy, retinitis pigmentosa, incomplete cleft lip, short stature (less than third percentile), mild delay in development, and seizures. To date, no etiology or pathogenetic mechanism has been discovered to account for these, and no similar cases have been encountered in the literature.

ACKNOWLEDGMENTS

We would like to acknowledge the help of many individuals in the study of this patient, particularly Drs. B. Boulton, W. J. Tze, A. MacDonald, and B. J. Wood. This study was supported in part by Medical Research Council of Canada, grant No. MA 4539

S. L. Yong
R. B. Lowry
J. E. Jan

C — RING 13 CHROMOSOME ASSOCIATED WITH MICROCEPHALY, CONGENITAL HEART DEFECT, INTRAUTERINE GROWTH RETARDATION, AND ABNORMAL SKIN PIGMENTATION

A number of reports have been published dealing with the phenotype of patients with a ring 13 or with a deletion of the long arm of chromosome 13. We report a ring 13 case with striking pigmentary changes in the skin.

The patient was born in 1974, the only child of this union. The father is reported to have a normal daughter by a different spouse. There is no consanguinity and at the time of the proband's birth the father was 26 and the mother 23 years old. The father had hyperuricemia and gouty nephropathy as did his father and grandfather.

One month before conception an unknown quantity of LSD was taken by the mother; about 2 weeks before conception she had a smallpox vaccination and polio inoculation. Maternal weight gain was about 7 kg and fetal movements reduced. At 1 week of gestation she had a fever (39.5°C) for which she was not treated; the remainder of the pregnancy was uneventful. The presentation and delivery at 41 weeks were normal. Birthweight was 2,353 gm, length 47 cm and head circumference 30 cm. The skin was reported to be normal at birth and there were no episodes of vesicles or bullae. Pigmentation was noted sometime in the first month of life, and subsequently a heart murmur, slow development, and growth retardation were noted. He sat at 8 months, crawled at 11 months, and at 18 months was beginning to stand and walk with support. He had no words.

Examination

At 18 months he had psychomotor and growth retardation. Head circumference was 42.1 cm (less than 3rd percentile), height 79 cm (10th percentile) and weight (at 15 months) 7.5 kg (less than 3rd percentile). There were bilateral epicanthic folds, upward slanting palpebral fissures (Fig. 1), and an intermittent esophoria. The ears were large but normal in shape and position with no rotation. Teeth, mouth and palate were normal. An ejection systolic murmur was noted and thought to be due to a small ventriculoseptal defect or minor

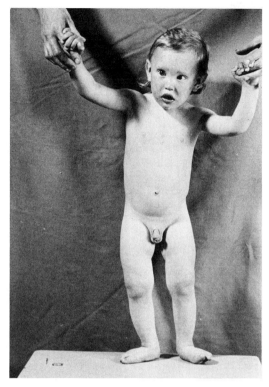

Fig. 1. Shows generally normal phenotype with upward slanting palpebral fissures, epicanthic folds, large ears, prominent, open lips, left esophoria, severe planovalgus feet and pigmentation on the chest.

degree of pulmonary stenosis. The femoral pulses were palpable and blood pressure was 90/70 mm Hg. There was no enlargement of liver or spleen and the genitalia were normal with both testes in the scrotum. The cranial nerves appeared normal apart from some facial asymmetry with the right side appearing to move less well than the left. There were no cataracts or colobomata, and the optic disks were normal. Tone was diminished; however, power in the limbs was normal. There was no clonus. Plantar reflexes were flexor and the other deep tendon reflexes were present although those in the left arm were more brisk than in the right. There was normal absence of the Moro, grasp, and asymmetric tonic neck reflexes and the parachute response was normal. Placing responses were absent and the Landau response was diminished. On the Gesell assessment (CA 18 months), he was able to complete most of the items at the 40-week level, while at the 52-week level, he had about half of the items. He had an occasional

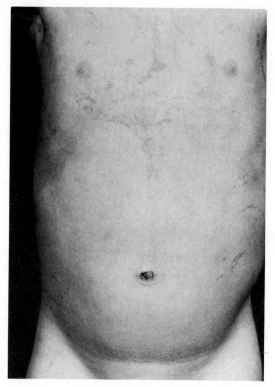

Fig. 2. Anterior chest and abdomen showing patches of abnormal pigmentation.

15-month level item. Language, however, was at the 28-week level. He could walk with support. The hands and feet were normal except for a left simian crease. There were striking patches of brown pigmentation on the skin, mainly on the trunk front and back (Figs. 2 and 3). Those on the back were in a linear swirling pattern. There were also two areas of depigmentation. Scalp hair was normal.

Investigations

Dermatoglyphics

	1	2	3	4	5	<atd	Simian Crease	Hallucals
R	Lu·	A	Lu	Lr	Lu	52°	—	LD
L	Lu	Lu	Lr	Lu	Lu	60°	+	LD

Urinary amino acid chromatogram was normal. Screening test for mucopolysaccharides was negative. Electroencephalogram (EEG) was within

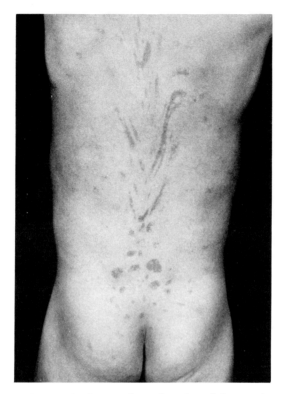

Fig. 3. Posterior view showing linear and round patches of pigmentation plus an area of depigmentation to the left.

normal limits. Roentgenogram of skull confirmed microcephaly but was otherwise unremarkable. Skeletal maturation was within normal limits. Skin biopsy
of the pigmented lesion showed mild hyperkeratosis with prominent melanin
pigmentation of the cells along the basal layer and melanin pigment within
histiocytes; biopsy findings were not diagnostic of incontinentia pigmenti.

Chromosome analysis from Giemsa-banded preparations revealed that one of the
number 13 chromosomes was in the form of a ring [46,XY,r (13) (p13 q34)]
(Fig. 4). Since nearly all the bands of chromosome 13 are visible in the ring
(Fig. 5), the break points on the chromosome were probably in the satellite
region (p13) and near the distal end of the long arm (q34). Evidence that much
of the 13p arm is present in the ring was provided by the occasional observation
of "satellite" association between the ring and other D-group chromosomes.
The ring chromosome was present in all cells observed and about 5% of the cells
had a dicentric ring. No cells had minute rings, quadricentric rings, or inter-
locking rings. All other chromosomes of the karyotype appeared normal. It was
not possible to obtain parental chromosomes.

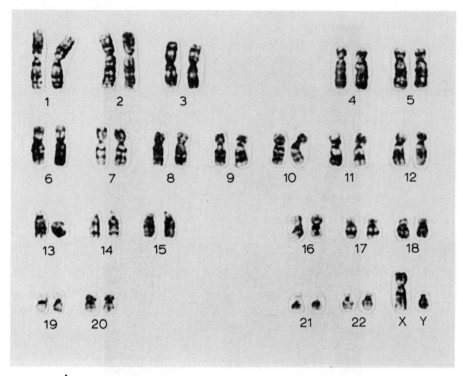

Fig. 4. The karyotype of the patient showing the ring 13 chromosome [46, XY, r(13) (p13 q34)].

Comment

Holmes et al [1] and Fried et al [2] have delineated some of the phenotypic features seen in ring 13 syndrome. Our patient shows many of them: microcephaly, intrauterine growth retardation, epicanthic folds, upward slanting palpebral fissures, and large ears; however, to our knowledge none have been described with such striking pigmentation. At first sight this suggested incontinentia pigmenti, but there was no history of prior vesicle formation and the distribution and biopsy findings were not in favor of that diagnosis. In addition, the patient lacked the ocular, dental and scalp hair manifestations of incontinentia pigmenti. Whether the immediate events prior to conception, ie LSD, smallpox vaccination and poliomyelitis inoculation, have anything to do with the product of a ring chromosome remains speculative.

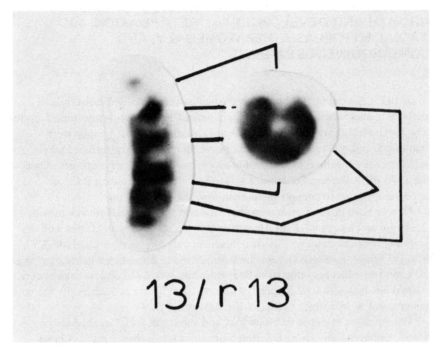

Fig. 5. The ring 13 with its normal homolog showing presence of all the G-dark bands. Lines indicate homologous bands.

ACKNOWLEDGMENTS

We would like to thank the following for help in studying this patient: Drs. K. O. Asante, H. Patel, M. W. Patterson, J. A. Pratt-Johnson, and W. J. Sands. These studies were supported in part by the Medical Research Council of Canada, grant No. MA 4539.

REFERENCES

1. Holmes LB, Moser HB, Halldorsson S, Mack C, Pant SS, Matzilevich B: "Mental Retardation: An Atlas of Disease With Associated Physical Abnormalities." New York: MacMillan, 1972, pp 168–169.
2. Fried K, Rosenblatt M, Mundel G, Krikler R: Ring chromosome 13 syndrome. Clin Genet 7:203–208, 1975.

R. B. Lowry
F. J. Dill

D — "ALDOLASE A" DEFICIENCY WITH SYNDROME OF GROWTH AND DEVELOPMENTAL RETARDATION, MID-FACIAL HYPOPLASIA, HEPATOMEGALY, AND CONSANGUINEOUS PARENTS

In 1973, Beutler et al [1] reported a new syndrome of red cell aldolase deficiency and hemolytic anemia. Their patient had many dysmorphic features, and psychomotor and growth retardation. No clinical photographs were published, and the title of their publication precluded easy retrieval when searching for congenital malformation or dysmorphogenetic syndromes. Since the 1976 Birth Defects Conference was to be held in Vancouver, B.C., an opportunity arose to present the patient since he resided there.

He was born in 1968 after a normal full-term pregnancy. Birthweight was 2,240 gm and length 43.2 cm. He was noted to have an unusual facies, and dry and very lax skin; however, his chromosomes were apprently normal (46,XY). At 4 weeks of age, he began to have loose stools and at 6 weeks his hematocrit was 20% and reticulocyte count 10%. Red and white blood cell structure appeared normal but platelets were reduced in number. The liver was 4 cm below the costal margin, and he had slight edema of the legs, and ascites.

There was no evidence of blood loss, and the stools were negative for occult blood. Urinalysis was normal. Serum bilirubin was less than 1 mg%. A bone marrow test showed hyperactive cellularity with no evidence of malignancy.

Further Laboratory Investigations

Results of urine amino acid and mucopolysaccharide screening were normal. PBI was 7.6 μg%. Alkaline phosphatase 606 IU; thymol turbidity 2.5 units, serum proteins 4.3—4.8 gm%. Serologic tests for toxoplasmosis, histoplasmosis, and syphilis were negative. Repeated fasting blood sugars were determined using a glucose oxidase method. The lowest value was 54.5 mg%, and the highest, 66 mg%. Glucagon stimulation did not raise the fasting blood sugar. There was no hematuria or melena on numerous examinations. The Coombs test was negative and no cold agglutinins were detected. Hematocrit remained at 40% with a reticulocyte response varying from 3—16%.

Futher Progress

Because of the possibility of a hepatoblastoma, an open biopsy was decided and laparotomy performed. The liver was enlarged, smooth and firm, and the spleen was normal size. Microscopic examination of the liver disclosed fairly wide bands of fibrous tissue infiltrated by small numbers of chronic inflammatory cells to form a meshwork dividing the liver tissue. Within the bands there was

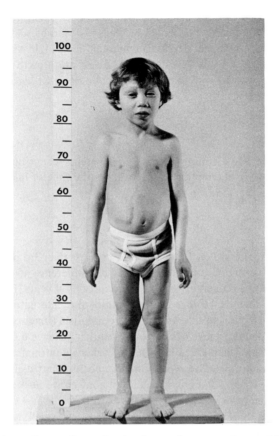

Fig. 1. At age 7 years, 8 months, showing small stature and general features.

considerable excess of bile ducts but no significant abnormality of the vascular system. No evidence of significant bile stasis was noted. The boundary between the fibrous bands and the liver cells was clearly demarcated in almost all areas with the liver cells arranged in an orderly manner and no evidence of an abnormal vascular system. The liver cells were noted to contain moderate amounts of sudanophilic lipid and were heavily laden with glycogen. There was no significant extramedullary hematopoiesis. The feature of fibrosis was consistent with congenital hepatic fibrosis, but the possibility of a glycogen storage disease was still considered. A frozen specimen of liver was sent to Professor Hers in Belgium. Initial findings suggested Type 6 glycogen storage disease. A fructose tolerance test was performed and a rise in blood glucose was obtained, demonstrating that there was no lack of glucose-6-phosphatase.

The family moved from England to Canada and subsequent investigation in Winnipeg and Duarte revealed that both red cells and fibroblasts were deficient in adolase A activity. (Further details can be found in [1]). It is of interest to note that parental adolase A levels were normal. The patient's growth and development have always been slow; he walked at 2 years, spoke single words at 4 years, and sentences at 7 years.

Family History

The parents were first cousins, all four grandparents were from Roumania. The father was 24 and the mother 23 years old at the time of his birth. No other similar cases were known in the family.

Examination

At 7 years, 8 months (Fig. 1): height 97.5 cm (less than 3rd percentile), weight 13.5 kg (less than 3rd percentile), head circumference 45 cm (less than 2nd percentile). Developmental age was approximately 4 years. Facies (Figs. 2 and 3) — flat midface with low nasal bridge and epicanthic folds, alternating strabismus, mild ptosis, telangiectasis of lids, and mild hypotelorism (inner canthal distance 2.2 cm, interpupillary distance 4.3 cm, outer canthal distance 6.6 cm — all less than 3rd percentile). The teeth, although small, showed normal mixed dentition and the palate was normal. Ears were normal in position but slightly cup-shaped. There was a low posterior hairline with a short nonwebbed neck. A grade 2–3/6 systolic ejection murmur was heard. The liver was palpable at 4 cm below the costal margin, and there was no splenomegaly. Penis was small, testes were descended. Neurologic examination was unremarkable. Musculoskeletal system joints were slightly loose and there was slight syndactyly of toes 2 and 3 bilaterally. The skin was dry, thin, and slightly hyperelastic with a prominent venous pattern; fingernails were very short (Fig. 4).

Investigations

Repeat chromosome studies including Giemsa banding disclosed no abnormalities. Skeletal roentgenograms showed microcephaly, hypoplasia of the maxilla, overtubulated, delicate appearing long bones, large cuboid bones, horizontally directed sacrum, and mildly delayed bone age (6 year level). Studies of growth hormone disclosed no deficiency. The patient has continued to have evidence of a hemolytic anemia. A recent restudy by Beutler (personal communication, 1976) confirmed the deficiency of aldolase A.

Dermatoglyphic examination showed that there were whorl patterns on all 10 digits. Both axial triradii were in the t^i position and there was no clinodactyly or

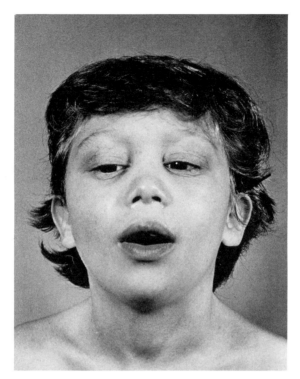

Fig. 2. Note ptosis, epicanthic folds, hypotelorism, flat midface, and slightly cup-shaped ears.

simian creases. Both hallucal patterns were whorl. Parental dermatoglyphics have not been obtained.

COMMENT

Since aldolase A is found in muscle, red cells, and also in brain it seems reasonable to conclude that the enzyme deficiency is responsible for this dysmorphogenetic syndrome. In describing the phenotype complete with photographs, we are hopeful that others may identify similar cases. The presence of an enzyme defect, together with the consanguinity, increases the likelihood of this syndrome being an autosomal recessive trait, but makes it also possible that the boy may be homozygous at two or more recessive loci. Since inborn errors of metabolism are not usually associated with malformations, the boy's dysmorphogenetic syndrome may represent homozygosity of gene(s) not responsible for the aldolase deficiency.

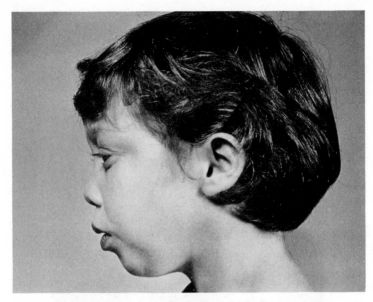

Fig. 3. Note flat midface, mildly receding jaw, low hairline, and short neck.

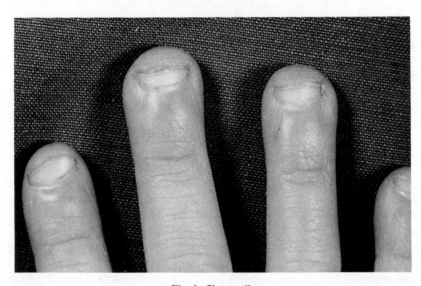

Fig. 4. Short nails.

TABLE 1.

Intermediate	Patient	Patient's mother	Normal values	Patients with reticulocytosis
G 6 P	43.40	37.40	30.5 ± 5.3	61.
F 6 P	13.32	6.73	9.6 ± 1.5	22.0
FDP	25.85	2.17	2.1 ± 0.3	3.0
DHAP	18.95	9.46	10.5 ± 1.4	18.2
2–PGA	42.69	43.63	56.7 ± 5.5	60.7
3–PGA	7.27	5.59	5.5 ± 1.4	10.7
PEP	16.10	11.18	11.6 ± 2.0	20.1
Pyruvate	67.9	47.4	56.3 ± 8.8	68.6
Lactate	913.7	830.3	964 ± 132	1103
ATP	1286	1321	1438 ± 99	
2,3 DPG	3347	2842	4171 ± 36	

All values are expressed as μMoles/ml RBC except for lactate and pyruvate, which are in μMoles/ml whole blood. From Ernest Beutler, Division of Medicine, City of Hope National Medical Center, Duarte, California.

ACKNOWLEDGMENTS

The authors would like to acknowledge the assistance of the following in studying this patient: Drs. E. Beutler, M. Patterson, D. W. Smith, J. Hall, B. D. Hall, P. Baird, P. M. MacLeod, B. MacGillivray, S. Wood, and Miss L. K. Suderman.

This work was supported in part by Medical Research Council of Canada grant No. MA 4539.

REFERENCES

1. Beutler E, Scott S, Bishop A, Margolis N, Matsumoto F, Kuhl W: Red cell aldolase deficiency and hemolytic anemia: A new syndrome. Trans Assoc Am Physicians 76:154–166, 1973.

COMMENT by Dr. E. Beutler

Our original studies of this case were necessarily limited, since the family was living in Canada, and samples had to be shipped to us for study. We were very pleased, therefore, when the patient was brought to Southern California for a family vacation, and we had an opportunity to carry out studies which could only be conducted on fresh blood cells. His reticulocyte count was only 1.9%, and the activity of hexokinase was only slightly increased, to 2.13 U/gm Hb (normal = 1.27 ± 0.18 U/gm Hb). These findings indicate that hemolysis was quite mild at this time. The level of red cell intermediates is summarized in Table 1. The ratio of fructose diphosphate (FDP) to dihydroxyacetone phosphate (DHAP) was increased. This is consistent with the location of the metabolic block at the aldolase step. $^{14}CO_2$ evolution from ^{14}C-1 glucose was at the upper limit, at 2.6 nMoles/ml RBC/min. In our earlier studies, peculiarities in the results of some of our assays led us to the conclusion that increased blood glyceraldehyde might be present. However, examination of fresh blood, obtained either in the fasting state or 1.5 hr after loading with 1 gm of fructose/kg body weight failed to reveal the presence of glyceraldehyde.

To date, we know of no other cases of aldolase A deficiency. However, it is hoped that Drs. Lowry and Hanson's report will draw attention to the unusual phenotype associated with this enzyme defect, and that other cases may come to light.

R. B. Lowry
J. W. Hanson

Selected Abstracts

FATAL NEPHROSIS, HYDROCEPHALUS, THIN SKIN, BLUE SCLERAS, GROWTH RETARDATION AND CHARACTERISTIC FACIES IN TWO BROTHERS: CLINICAL, STRUCTURAL AND BIOCHEMICAL STUDIES

D. L. Daentl, C. F. Piel, R. C. Siegle, J. Townsend, D. W. Wara, C. Gooding, and R. Bachmann

Departments of Growth and Development, Pediatrics, Medicine and Neuropathology, University of California, San Francisco and The Permanente Medical Group, Oakland, California

An unusual renal disease which was fatal at approximately age three years has afflicted two brothers of normal intellect who also had hydrocephalus, strikingly similar facies with narrowed mid-dimension, generalized thin skin with sparse blond hair, eyebrows and lashes, blue scleras and severe growth retardation.

Onset of the renal disease occurred at age one and a half years, beginning with proteinuria which became progressively more severe until renal failure occurred. The terminal course of the younger brother was accelerated by severe hypertension which was resistant to control and associated with high plasma renin levels. An unequal kidney size in this boy was due to failure of the left kidney to grow. The most striking electron microscopic feature found in the renal biopsy of this boy's right kidney was widespread irregular translucent thickening on the glomerular endothelial surface of the basement membrane. In addition, there was deposition of electron dense material in the subepithelial surface of the basement membrane and coalescence of the foot processes of the epithelium.

In both boys the postmortem brain examination resulted in similar findings. There was downward displacement of the cerebellar tonsils and descent of the vermis and medulla through the foramen magnum without the presence of a meningomyelocele or fixation of the spinal cord.

An additional post mortem finding was T-cell depletion in the thymus and lymph nodes. However, cellular immunodeficiency was not detectable during life.

Marked thinning of the scleras was the only pathologic finding in the eyes. The connective tissue of the skin was also diminished in amount and, viewed in

Birth Defects: Original Article Series, Volume XIII, Number 3B, pages 229–264
© 1977 The National Foundation

the electron microscope, the numbers of collagen fibers were reduced.

Biochemical studies of collagen composition and synthesis are in progress and preliminary findings suggest that there may be unusual amino acid composition of extracted collagen. Although a collagen abnormality could account for some of the clinical findings, no unifying hypothesis can yet be advanced to explain the basis of all features of the syndrome.

GROWTH FAILURE, CLEFT PALATE, ECTODERMAL DYSPLASIA AND APPARENT PANCREATIC INSUFFICIENCY —? A NEW SYNDROME

M. A. Donlan

Inland Empire Genetics Counseling Clinic, Deaconess Hospital, Spokane, Washington

A brother and sister with evidence of posterior (soft) palate clefts, relative micrognathia, growth failure, and apparent associated pancreatic insufficiency are described. The oldest child, a girl is now four and a half years of age. She was born as an uncomplicated pregnancy to unrelated parents. The child was born as a term gestation, but had a birthweight of 5 lbs 2 oz. She had surgery for annular pancreas at two days of age at the Children's Orthopedic Hospital and Medical Center in Seattle, Washington. Duodenojejunostomy was performed. Subsequent to that time she has had severe growth retardation, and on further evaluation (in 1973) she was found to have absent stool trypsins. She was also evaluated for severe eczema. With the empiric addition of Viokase there was an improvement in her growth (which still remains far below the 3rd percentile). Growth hormone evaluation has been normal. The eczema has remained in good control, unless the enzyme is discontinued, at which time there is a clear-cut worsening of her eczema. Chromosome count (without banding) has been normal. Multiple sweat chloride determinations have been within normal limits.

The child's brother was born in 1974, again with an uncomplicated pregnancy. This child's birthweight was 6 lbs 11 oz, and the child developed evidence of respiratory obstruction shortly after birth. This child also had a posterior cleft palate, as well as relative micrognathia, and an endotracheal tube was put in place. The endotracheal tube was subsequently able to be removed and the child did not require further procedures, but was re-evaluated for failure to thrive at approximately three months of age. At that time this child also had evidence of trypsin deficiency on stool evaluation with again normal multiple repeat sweat chlorides. He has had significant failure to thrive and has also developed eczema. Ectodermal dysplasia is manifested by the thin skin in both children, as well as evidence of dental hypoplasia.

SAETHRE-CHOTZEN SYNDROME: A BROAD AND VARIABLE MALFORMATION PATTERN

J. M. Friedman, J. W. Hanson, and D. W. Smith

Department of Pediatrics, University of Washington, School of Medicine, Seattle, Washington

We report a family in which 15 members in 5 generations are affected to variable degrees with a consistent pattern of abnormalities. Craniofacial features include marked delay of fontanel closure, brachycephaly, high flat forehead, broad flat midface with small maxilla, prominent nose with broad triangular columella, mild blepharophimosis, labial pits at the corners of the mouth, and small ears. Hands and feet show mild soft tissue syndactyly, clinodactyly, mild camptodactyly, brachyphalangy and broad great toes. Less consistent features include mild mesomelic short stature, strabismus, supernumerary teeth and altered dermatoglyphics.

Radiographic features include hyperostosis of the frontal calvarium, mild hypoplasia of the distal portion of the clavicles and distal phalanges, and small iliac wings.

Although craniosynostosis is either lacking or relatively mild in affected members of this family, their features are otherwise strikingly similar to those of patients with the Saethre-Chotzen syndrome. This family demonstrates that the Saethre-Chotzen syndrome is a broad pattern of craniofacial and other skeletal malformations in which craniosynostosis may sometimes occur.

TRISOMY 12p, A CLINICALLY RECOGNIZABLE SYNDROME

O. S. Alfi and M. Lange

Division of Medical Genetics, Childrens Hospital of Los Angeles, University of Southern California School of Medicine, Los Angeles, California

A 7-year-old female with a paternal karyotype 46,XX,der(14), t(12;14) (p11; p11) is reported. The clinical features, when compared to the 3 cases reported

in the literature, presented a distinctive phenotype. The general craniofacial structure had a unique appearance. There was a relatively large head with a prominent
high forehead. The facial profile was flat. The midface was short and appeared compressed. The bigonial diameter was the widest part of the face giving the appearance of a puffy masseteric region. The chin was fleshy and square. The abnormal
facial features included thick and irregular insertions of the eyebrows, almond-
shaped horizontal eyes, short narrow nose, malar flattening, thin upper lip, everted
lower lip, irregularly spaced teeth, and small ears with rolled helix, prominent
anthelix and deep concha. The neck was short and the trunk was long in comparison to the limbs. Unusual vertical creases were present over the metacarpol-
phalangeal joints and the terminal phalanges were shortened with short 5th finger
and thumb. The feet were also unusual. The toes were short with polysyndactyly
of the great toe and a prominent heel. Genu valgus and talus valgus deformities
were also noted. This patient was functioning in the severely retarded range.
When this case is compared to the 3 cases in the literature a distinctive dysmorphic picture emerges. The main features that characterize all 4 cases of 12p
trisomy include the hourglass-shaped face with high forehead, compressed midface and wide bigonial diameter, almond-shaped eyes, short nose, everted lower
lip, abnormally shaped ears, and dimpling or furrows over the knuckles.

FAMILIAL AGENESIS OF THE CORPUS CALLOSUM WITH SPINAL CORD INVOLVEMENT: A NEW AUTOSOMAL RECESSIVE SYNDROME ORIGINATING IN CHARLEVOIX COUNTY

E. Andermann, F. Andermann, S. Carpenter, G. Karpati, A. Eisen, D. Melancon,
and J. Bergeron

Department of Neurology and Neurosurgery, Montreal Neurological Hospital and Institute,
McGill University and Department of Demography, University of Montreal, Montreal,
Quebec, Canada

In recent years, we have recognized a syndrome in French Canadian patients
originating from Charlevoix County who present with psychomotor retardation
and slowly progressive flaccid quadriparesis, most marked in the lower limbs.
Other features of the syndrome include brachycephaly, bilateral ptosis, strabismus, asymmetric facies, hypoplastic maxilla, large angle of the mandible, high-
arched palate, kyphoscoliosis, pigeon-chest deformities, and various digital
anomalies.

These patients have been proved to have complete agenesis of the corpus callosum, at times associated with heterotopia. The electrophysiologic findings indicated evidence for anterior horn cell disease. There was also a total absence of

sensory evoked potentials, which are considered to reflect involvement of the dorsal root ganglion. Gastrocnemius muscle biopsies showed denervation atrophy. By phase microscopy on semithin epon sections, sural nerves showed absence of almost all large myelinated fibers with preservation of small myelinated fibers and unmyelinated fibers. Wallerian degeneration was absent.

This combination of central and peripheral abnormalities is inherited as an autosomal recessive disorder, with remarkable intra- and interfamilial similarities. The syndrome has now been ascertained in 42 patients from 21 sibships. To date, 18 patients in 10 sibships have been examined. All the families originated from settlements between Baie St. Paul and La Malbaie, and most of the sibships have now been traced to a common ancestral couple who married in Quebec City in 1657.

Because of its high incidence this syndrome represents a major public health problem in Charlevoix County, as well as in the areas to which these families have migrated. Since carrier detection is not yet feasible by biochemical or morphologic means, genetic counseling with avoidance of consanguineous marriages is the only effective form of prevention. Although there have been a few isolated case reports of familial agenesis of the corpus callosum in the world literature, to our knowledge, the above syndrome has not been described elsewhere.

A SYNDROME OF COLLAGEN VASCULAR DISEASE, SPASTICITY AND MENTAL RETARDATION IN A FRENCH CANADIAN KINDRED

E. Andermann, I. E. Leppik, F. Andermann, A. H. Eisen, G. Karpati, S. Carpenter, L. Goldin, and R. C. Elston

Department of Neurology and Neurosurgery, Montreal Neurological Hospital and Institute, McGill University, Montreal, Quebec and Genetics Laboratory, Department of Biostatistics, School of Public Health, University of Nortn Carolina, Chapel Hill, North Carolina

We have ascertained 13 individuals in four sibships who exhibit a spectrum of clinical manifestations consisting of various forms of collagen vascular disease (CV) including discoid lupus, polymyositis, dermatomyositis, and juvenile rheumatoid arthritis; mild spastic paraplegia with mild mental retardation (SP); and severe spastic quadriplegia with severe mental retardation (SQ) alone or in combination: CV (2); probable CV (2); CV + SP (4); SP (2); SQ (3). All 13 affected individuals come from a small fishing village in the Gaspé peninsula and are offspring of consanguineous marriages. Their parents can all be traced to a common ancestral couple of Acadian descent.

The apparently random combination of manifestations in this closely inbred kindred might suggest that at least two autosomal recessive traits, those for CV and for SP/SQ, are segregating independently. However, linkage studies on 34 family members using 23 independent systems resulted in significant linkage with the Duffy locus ($p < 0.05$) when all phenotypes were considered together. HL-A typing in one sibship showed that all affected individuals inherited at least one W21 gene, regardless of phenotype. Furthermore, all affected individuals and their parents had significantly elevated IgA levels. Thus, the possibility of a single mutant gene with pleiotropic effects, perhaps determining a common immunologic defect responsible for both the collagen vascular and neurologic manifestations, seems more likely. Although familial instances of collagen vascular disease have been described in the literature, to our knowledge, a syndrome of collagen vascular disease with mental retardation and spasticity has not.

HYPERSENSITIVE FURROWED MOUTH AND ELEVATED SALIVA IgE: A NEW SYNDROME

J. A. Anderson, C. E. Jackson, S. Yanari, E. A. Krull, and I. Magdea

Departments of Medicine and Dermatology, Henry Ford Hospital, Detroit, Michigan

Three patients in 2 families are described and compared with a case previously reported by Huntley et al (South Med J 63:917, 1970) as an allergic protein-losing gastroenteropathy. All four cases were severely atopic, especially to foods, and had eczema, allergic rhinitis, and asthma. Multiple episodes of angioedema of the mouth occurred with food ingestion at an early age. At about 5 years of age chronic changes occurred in the tongue, lips, and buccal mucosa in each of the four cases. In one case, the process extended to the upper third of the esophagus. In the case described by Huntley et al, the process involved the entire gastrointestinal tract. These chronic changes were characterized by edema, fissures, and furrows of the mucosa with the appearance not unlike that seen in congenital scrotal tongue. In the case described by Huntley et al, the child had a severe protein-losing enteropathy and hypersecretion of saliva. In that case and one of ours, chronic salivary gland enlargement was observed. In two of the four cases shortness of stature was noted. Serum and salivary IgE levels were studied in members of these two families and in the case reported by Huntley et al. Elevated serum levels (68,000-23,000 u/ml) were found in each of the 4 cases along with elevated levels in unconcentrated saliva (12-104 u/100 gm albumin). Serum IgE: salivary IgE ratios were 340:1, 192:1, 354:1, and 1,667:1. IgE was undetectable in saliva of patients with hay fever, food-stimulated hives, angioedema, and congenital scrotal tongue, and in normal individuals with serum IgE levels <1,000 units. In five selected atopic patients with serum IgE of 1,000-9,500, up to 3 units of IgE were found in 10X concentrated saliva (serum/saliva IgE ratio of 3,100:1). Mucosal biopsies of the patients with hypersensitive furrowed mouth were characterized by intracellular edema, plasma cells, eosinophils, and lymphocytes. In the one family with a girl and her mother affected with the furrowed mouth condition, one of three maternal aunts and the maternal grandfather had elevated salivary IgE levels. In the other family only one child had the furrowed mouth condition even though two of three sibs and the father had elevated salivary IgE levels. Postulating the salivary IgE elevation to be a dominant trait allows estimation of possible linkage relationships of the gene for this condition and that for HL-A (1 recombinant in 10 informative sibs). Further studies in such families will be needed to elucidate the mechanism for the furrowed mouth syndrome, its relationship to immunoglobulins, and the exact mode of inheritance.

DELETION OF THE SHORT ARM OF CHROMOSOME 18— A SYNDROME?

E. C. Bond, K. Chang, and S. McDonald

Department of Medical Sciences, Southern Illinois University, School of Medicine, Springfield, Illinois

A case with a translocation between chromosomes 18 and 22 resulting in a deletion of the short arm of chromosome 18 is presented and the clinical picture is compared with Noonan syndrome and Turner syndrome. Growth and mental-motor retardation, broad-bridged nose, receding chin, ptosis, hypertelorism, antimongoloid slant, large and low-set ears, broad mouth with a downward slant, prominent dental malformation and caries, pectus excavatum, and retarded bone age are the most usual findings.

AUTOSOMAL RECESSIVE MICROCEPHALY ASSOCIATED WITH CHORIORETINOPATHY

J. M. Cantú, A. Rojas, R. Fragoso, D. Garcia-Cruz, and C. Manzano

Instituto Mexicano del Seguro Social, México, D.F., México

McKusick et al have described eight cases of microcephaly observed in two sibships of an inbred group (Arch Ophthalmol 75:597, 1966). In addition to the usual features of microcephaly they have observed chorioretinal dysplasia in all the affected individuals suggesting that the association could indicate the existence of an entity different from simple autosomal recessive microcephaly.

A similar condition has been seen recently in sibs (one boy and two girls). The consanguineous parents and 3 other sibs were normal. In all affected cases, intrauterine environmental etiologic factors (x rays, toxoplasmosis, cytomegalovirus) which can lead to a similar syndrome, were investigated with negative results. Based on these observations, it seems clear that a distinct form of autosomal recessive microcephaly associated with chorioretinopathy can be separated from the heterogeneous state of microcephaly.

A SYNDROME OF PECULIAR FACIES, FIRM AURICULAR APPENDAGES, BLUE SCLERAS, AND GENERAL HYPOTONIA: A NEW SYNDROME?

F. Char and J. H. Bornhofen

Department of Pediatrics, University of Arkansas School of Medicine, Little Rock, Arkansas

The purpose of this communication is to report a new syndrome consisting of firm auricular appendages, blue scleras, general hypotonia, and peculiar facies.

The patient, a 2.5-year-old while male, was born in 1974. He was the second child of nonconsanguineous parents. The father was 30 years old and the mother 26 years old at the time of the patient's birth. The pregnancy was uneventful. There was no history of maternal drug use or illnesses.

Family history: The patient's father has a history of slow motor development. He began to walk at age 1.5 years with support and drooled until he was approximately 3 to 4 years old. He has speech difficulty. He has always had humpback and is said to have had "polio." He had plastic surgery in early infancy for his abnormal ears to "free them from the head." He had a tenth grade education and is of average intelligence, presently working in a copper plant. No others in the family are similarly affected. The patient has one sister, age 6 years, who is normal.

Physical examination: Height 81 cm; weight 9.95 kg; head circumference 48 cm. The fontanels were closed. The facies was peculiar. The forehead was high. The lips were full. The scleras were blue. Funduscopic examination was normal. The ears were firm and auricles were almost completely attached to the head and were somewhat low set. The palate was high arched. The lungs were clear. There was a grade II systolic murmur localized in the 4th left intercostal space. The ribs appeared somewhat flared. The abdominal musculature was laxed. No masses were palpable. There was generalized hypotonia. Deep tendon reflexes were normal. He could crawl on elbows and knees. He could not stand. He could say 2 to 3 words. Personal-social behavior appeared to be normal for age.

Nerve conduction velocity of the right peroneal nerve was 40 m/sec with a terminal latency of 2.6 m/sec; these values were normal. EMI scan was normal except for a scaphoid cranium. Blood chemistries were normal. Chromosome studies showed 46,XY.

Physical examination of the patient's father showed frontal prominence, small chin, full lower lip, and firm auricles which were not pliable. The scleras were blue. Funduscopic examination was normal. There was marked thoracic kyphosis. Muscle tone was within normal limits. Tendon reflexes were normal.

FETAL HYDANTOIN SYNDROME ASSOCIATED WITH TURNER SYNDROME

H. Chen, J. Perrin, R. Wesley, and P. V. Woolley, Jr.

Department of Pediatrics, Children's Hospital of Michigan and Wayne State University, Detroit, Michigan

Fetal hydantoin syndrome seen in children born to epileptic mothers treated with diphenylhydantoin anticonvulsants during pregnancy has recently been delineated. The syndrome consists of a broad, multisystem pattern of abnormalities including craniofacial anomalies, nail and digital hypoplasia, prenatal-onset growth deficiency, and mental deficiency. Noonan syndrome and Coffin-Siris syndrome have sometimes been confused with this pattern of malformation. However, Turner syndrome has not been noted to be associated. We wish to report here a case of unusual combination of the fetal hydantoin syndrome and Turner syndrome.

The propositus, a 4-month-old female, was born to a 22-year-old gravida 1 para 1 mother after full-term pregnancy with a birthweight of 2,325 gm and birthlength of 44.4 cm. The mother has grand mal seizures and received 300 mg of diphenylhydantoin and 100 mg phenobarbital daily throughout this pregnancy. The mother had 3 seizures during the first and second trimester.

The patient is a poor nibbler and fails to gain weight. Her malformations include growth deficiency, microcephaly, marked epicanthal folds, broad and depressed nasal bridge, short nose with upturned nostrils, wide mouth with prominent maxilla and lips, short neck with wrinkled skin, low-set ears, coarse hair, distally displaced nipples, cubitus valgus, hypoplasia of nails and distal phalanges, and increased digital arches. Chromosome analysis of cultured lymphocytes showed a 45,XO karyotype.

Association of Turner syndrome and the fetal hydantoin syndrome in this case is probably fortuitous. Turner syndrome, however, should be included in the differential diagnosis in view of this case report and the similarity of malformation pattern of the fetal hydantoin syndrome with Noonan syndrome, especially in the female; whether chromosomal nondisjunction in this case is related to teratogenetic effect of hydantoin is unknown.

BLOOM-LIKE SYNDROME WITH UNUSUAL SKELETAL ANOMALIES

H. Chen, A. K. Poznanski, and P. V. Woolley, Jr.

Children's Hospital of Michigan and Wayne State University, Detroit, Michigan

The propositus, a 12-year-old boy of Italian and German descent, presented clinically with dwarfism, malar hypoplasia, and congenital telangiectatic erythema which worsened with exposure to light. His phenotype resembled Bloom syndrome but he had less severe dwarfism, milder telangiectatic erythema, splenomegaly, and skeletal anomalies. However, cytogenetic studies on the blood sample, kindly performed by Dr. James German, New York, revealed no increase in the number of sister chromatic exchanges in phytohemagglutinin-stimulated lymphocytes.

The hands and feet are characterized by increased density of many of the epiphyses, particularly of the middle and distal phalanges. Some epiphyses are cone shaped. The entire carpus is diminished in size, occupying considerably less space than normal. There is a prominent pseudoepiphysis of the 2nd metacarpal and hallux deformity of the great toes. The skeletal age of 6 years was obtained at the chronologic age of 12 years. There is flattening and irregularity of the left femoral head suggesting Legg-Perthes disease and a single exostosis of the distal diaphysis of the right femur.

The bone changes seen in the hand roentgenograms are quite unusual but resemble the findings in epiphyseal dysplasias, particularly the presence of the small carpals and the dense epiphyses. The cone shape of the epiphysis, however, does not fit very well with this. Thiemann syndrome has some coning of the epiphysis and sclerosis, and the trichopharyngeal syndrome may be associated with cone and ivory epiphyses, and Legg-Perthes disease.

It will be fascinating to examine films on other patients with Bloom syndrome variants to determine if this is a consistent pattern or one simply related to this patient alone.

45,XO/46,XX/47,XX+18 MOSAICISM IN A FEMALE

C. Clark

Clinical Research Department, Alfred I. duPont Institute, Wilmington, Delaware

We describe mosaicism for 3 cell lines in a 5 8/12-year-old female, 45,XO/ 46,XX/47,XX+18. The mosaicism found in leukocytes cultured from peripheral blood is in the ratio of 47%-45,XO; 7%-46,XX; and 46%-XX+18. The prescence of 3 cell lines is verified by routine karyotyping and G-banded karyotyping. The findings of this laboratory are confirmed by M. A. Telfer, Ph.D. of Elwyn Institute.

Buccal smear preparations are negative for X-bodies. Dermatoglyphic findings are consistent with Turner syndrome despite the fact the ratio of the 47,XX+18 cell line to the 45,XO cell line is nearly equal. The dermatoglyphic patterns are in no way consistent with those reported for trisomy 18.

Our patient was initially seen in Child Diagnostic and Development Clinic because of mental retardation, slow development, and multiple congenital anomalies. She is the first born of 3 sibs. A 2 8/12-year-old male sib is being treated for early Blount disease. There is another male sib, aged 10 months, who has no apparent problems. The father was 18 years old and the mother was 20 years old at the time of birth of the proposita.

Ultimately, routine karyotyping, G-banding, and analyses from skin biopsies will be attained on the entire family in order to establish the origin of this very interesting mosaicism.

A SYNDROME OF DEGENERATIVE BONE DISEASE AND HEARING LOSS WITH AUTOSOMAL DOMINANT INHERITANCE

J. H. DiLiberti

Department of Pediatrics, University of Oregon Health Sciences Center, Portland, Oregon

Three children (ages 9,12, and 14 years) and their mother (age 32 years) were found to have a distinct group of abnormalities of the skeleton along with varying degrees of high frequency neural hearing loss. The maternal grandfather and great-grandfather are reported to have the same problems, but were not examined.

The following abnormalities were observed: 1) slipped capital femoral epiphyses or Legg-Perthes disease in 3 of 4 individuals examined; 2) hyperextensible fingers with "boutonniere" deformity in all 4 family members, with the same problem reported in other, presumably affected, individuals; 3) increased extension at the elbow with decreased supination; 4) high frequency neural hearing loss in all individuals; severe in the 3 children; 5) irregularities of the lumbar vertebral bodies with increasing severity with aging; 6) hallux valgus; 7) height greater than 97th percentile; 8) metaphyseal dysplasia.

Although several similarities with the Stickler syndrome are apparent there are several reasons for excluding that diagnosis: 1) complete lack of myopia or ocular problems in the pedigree; 2) absence of cleft palate and the Robin anomalad from the kindred; 3) lack of the prominent joints with arthropathy seen in the Stickler syndrome; 4) prominent abnormalities of the lumbar rather than thoracic spine; 5) absence of flat facies; 6) extremely tall stature; 7) metaphyseal dysplasia; 8) consistent phenotype in 4 generations.

This family appears to have a previously unreported dominantly inherited disorder of neural hearing loss and degenerative bone disease.

SAETHRE-CHOTZEN SYNDROME (SCS) WITH ADDITIONAL ABNORMALITIES IN A MEXICAN FAMILY

U. Francke, E. L. Gonzalez y Rivera, C. G. Delgado, and M. G. Ramos

Department of Pediatrics, University of California, San Diego, La Jolla, California and Unidad de Genetica Clinica, Hospital Infantil de Mexico, Mexico, D.F.

A Mexican man and 4 of his 6 children (3 male, 1 female, between the ages of 11 and 24 years) presented with a consistent and striking pattern of mostly craniofacial abnormalities. Craniosynostosis had led to a small head with flat forehead and decreased AP diameter, flat nasal bridge, and shallow orbits with proptosis of the eyes. The anterior hairline was low and extended down the cheeks in the preauricular area. They had various degrees of facial asymmetry and moderate-to-severe ptosis. There was maxillary hypoplasia, gothic palate, and crowding of teeth in the anterior upper segment with small or partially displaced lateral incisors. The noses were beaked with depressed tip and elongated nasal septum.

The following features involving soft tissue which have not been previously described in the SCS (Pantke et al, Birth Defects XI, No. 2, 190, 1975) were observed in this family: the edges of the eyelids were more or less irregular; the eyelashes were sparse medially, but heavy laterally, with an occasional double row; the external ears which were small and malformed had prominent unattached earlobes pointing anteriorly; there were deep furrows on the tongue.

The fingers were slightly short with distal tapering of the 1st and 2nd. There was no syndactyly. Two of the children had clinodactyly of the 5th finger. The feet were flat with wide spaces between the 1st and 2nd toes, and partial cutaneous syndactyly between the 2nd and 3rd.

Additional bony abnormalities included: short clavicles with prominent lateral ends; pectus excavatum; increased lumbar lordosis. The children had mild hearing loss; 2 of them had esotropia; all were of normal intelligence.

The responsible gene mutation is most likely autosomal dominant. It was fully expressed in all 5 affected individuals. There was no resemblance at all to unaffected family members. The father was the last born and the only affected member of a sibship of 7. His parents were reportedly unaffected. He appears to represent a new mutation, possibly related to increased paternal age.

GONADOBLASTOMA IN A CASE OF TURNER SYNDROME

W. M. Gooch, III, R. S. Wilroy, Jr., and R. L. Summitt

Departments of Pathology and Pediatrics, University of Tennessee Center for the Health Sciences, Memphis, Tennessee

This report describes a 13-year-old patient with the phenotypic features of Turner syndrome. Chromosomal analyses of multiple tissues revealed a presumptive mosaic karyotype, 45,X/46,X,mar. The cell line containing the marker chromosome constituted only a small minority of the cells analyzed. The marker chromosome was smaller than chromosomes of the G-group and was apparently acrocentric. The patient had no evidence of virilization, but she did experience thelarche and a few scant menstrual periods. She also had aortic stenosis and coarctation of the aorta. Approximately one year after repair of the coarctation the patient suddenly died as the result of an aortic aneurysm at the site of the coarctation repair.

Autopsy revealed that the breast enlargement was due to ductal hyperplasia without acinus formation. The patient had bilateral streak gonads, in each of which microscopic examination revealed gonadoblastoma. The neoplasm consisted of multiple aggregates of germ cells and immature Sertoli or granulosa cells. Hyaline bodies reminiscent of Call-Exner bodies were associated with the sex cord derivatives. Leydig cells or lutein cells were present in each gonad. Breast development is probably attributable to estrogen synthesis by the gonadoblastomata. The presence of gonadoblastomata in this patient suggests, even in the absence of masculinization, that the marker chromosome is a structurally abnormal Y chromosome.

A NEW SHORT-RIB POLYDACTYLY SYNDROME

J. Hall, M. Piepkorn, L. Karp, D. Hickok, and L. Wiegenstein

Department of Pediatrics, Medicine, Obstetrics, Gynecology and Pathology, University of Washington School of Medicine and the Children's Orthopedic Hospital, Seattle, Washington

Many different types of lethal neonatal dwarfism have been recognized. A recently delineated subgroup of lethal neonatal dwarfism is made up of the short-rib polydactyly syndromes. Two varieties are well described: 1) Saldino-Noonan and 2) Majewski. We have recently studied a neonate who appears to represent a third type of lethal short-rib polydactyly dwarfism.

The child was a 34-week stillborn, recognized to be abnormal one week before birth when roentgenograms were taken because of polyhydramnios. Pregnancy was otherwise normal and was the first pregnancy for 27-year-old parents. No family history of congenital malformations or consanguinity was known. Marked underossification was present in all bones except the base of the skull and clavicles. Ribs were short and relatively broad. No ossification of hands, feet, or lower limbs could be recognized. The child had markedly disproportionately small trunk and large head. Ocular hypertelorism and cleft palate were present. Limbs were flipper-like in appearance. Polysyndactyly was present in the hands. Three blob-shaped toes were present on each foot. Autopsy showed persistent left superior vena cava, hypoplastic respiratory tract, hypoplastic left kidney, bicornuate uterus, and absent right olfactory tract. Histologic studies of bone showed irregular endochondral plates. Electron microscopic studies showed accumulation of material resembling secretory products within chondrocytes.

A SYNDROME OF CRANIOFACIAL ANOMALIES, ECTODERMAL DEFECTS, AND CHONDROOSSEOUS DYSPLASIA WITH SIMILARITIES TO MELNICK-NEEDLES SYNDROME

J. W. Hanson, C. B. Graham, and J. G. Hall

Departments of Pediatrics and Radiology, University of Washington, School of Medicine, Seattle, Washington

We present a 7-year-old child with a bizarre syndrome born to normal unrelated parents. Craniofacial features include brachycephaly, frontal bossing, hypertelorism, optic nerve hypoplasia with abnormal retinal pigmentation, broad depressed nasal bridge, flat midface, cleft palate and alveolar ridge, and minor ear anomalies. The hair is sparse and fine, several teeth are missing, and the dental enamel is hypoplastic. The nails are thin and split by longitudinal fibrous ridges. A small focal area of dermal hypoplasia is present over the base of the nose. Limb abnormalities include symbrachydactyly, symphalangism, clinodactyly, metatarsus adductus, and bowing of long bones. Hydronephrosis was found shortly after birth. Growth has always been poor and mental performance may be slightly impaired.

Radiographic studies show a severe generalized chondroosseous dysplasia with some similarities to the Melnick-Needles syndrome. Mineralization is generally decreased with somewhat thinned tubular bone cortices. The skull is partially hyperostotic with shallow orbits and maxillary hypoplasia. Spinal segmentation anomalies with scoliosis and vertebral body collapse are prominent. The pelvis is small and dysplastic, and ribs show pronounced wavy variation in width. The long bones show diaphyseal cortical irregularity with old healed fractures. Only mild epiphyseal flattening and minimal metaphyseal changes are noted. Massive coalition of carpal and tarsal bones, metacarpal and metatarsal shortening, and symphalangism are present along with severe modeling defects of the phalanges.

7q DELETION SYNDROME?

E. L. Harris, R. S. Wappner, and C. G. Palmer

Departments of Medical Genetics and Pediatrics, Indiana University School of Medicine, Indianapolis, Indiana

A 5.5-year-old white girl with unusual facies and severe mental and physical retardation was found to have partial deletion of the long arm of chromosome 7. She was delivered at term after an uncomplicated pregnancy; birthweight was 2,900 gm. Severe feeding problems complicated the first 6 months of life. Markedly delayed developmental milestones and physical growth were noted from early infancy.

Physical examination revealed a slim, proportionately small-for-age, alert, friendly, white girl. Height was 87 cm, weight 9.32 kg, head circumference 43.5 cm; all parameters were approximately 5 standard deviations below the mean for age. The following physical findings were noted: prominent forehead, brachycephaly, prominent nose with bulbous tip, myopia, cupped simple helices of ears, bifid uvula, prominent labia, anal skin tags, hyperextensible joints, mild inversion of the feet with prominent heels, generalized decreased motor mass and tone without pathologic reflexes, and relatively lax skin—not redundant or thin. Developmental testing showed her to be functioning at a 12-month level. Dermatoglyphics were within normal limits. Chromosome studies with G (trypsin) and R (Giemsa) banding showed a deletion of the long arm of chromosome 7 del(7)(q32); 46,XX,del(7)(pter→q32:)].

Both parents had normal chromosomes. The only other pregnancy resulted in a spontaneous abortion at 4 months' gestation.

Review of the literature revealed only one other case of partial deletion of the long arm of chromosome 7 (Shokeir MHK et al: Clin Genet 4:360, 4:360, 1973). This report was of translocation of chromosomes 2 and 7 [+(2;7)]. The case resembled ours in body build, physical retardation, and abnormal ears. No other physical findings were found to be common to both cases.

ARTHROGRYPOSIS MULTIPLEX CONGENITA AND THE TURNER PHENOTYPE

I. Krieger

Department of Pediatrics, Wayne State University, Children's Hospital of Michigan, Detroit, Michigan

This symptom complex was described in 1972 (Am J Dis Child 123:141) by Krieger and Espiritu in 4 patients, including a pair of sibs. One of the 2 infants died; the other is currently 6 2/12 years old and the subject of this report because of previously unrecognized abnormalities.

The following findings were initially reported: mild linear growth failure, webbing of the neck with low posterior hairline, antimongoloid slant, high-arched palate, receding mandible, low-set ears, and broad forehead with supranasal prominence. This patient, like the other 3 of the original report, had flexion contractures of the elbows, wrists, interphalangeal joints, hips, knees, and ankles. Other abnormalities, that are frequently associated with arthrogryposis multiplex congenita, were: vertical talus and calcaneus varus, dimples over the radial head, scapula and sacroiliac joint, dislocation of the radial head, prominent xiphoid, syndactyly of the 4th and 5th toes, and excessive length of the 2nd and 3rd toes.

Contractures were also seen in the eyes and were recently recognized in the middle ears: The patient has the Stilling-Duane syndrome which consists of eye retraction with narrowing of the palpebral fissure on attempted adduction, and restricted abduction. Middle ear surgery at 3 10/12 years of age for conductive hearing loss revealed abnormalities of the head of the malleus and body of the incus. There was bony attachment of the malleus to the auditory canal with immobilization of the ossicular chain. The stapes and the oval and round windows were absent. A preauricular cyst and dermal sinus were removed. Corrective surgery of the hand and ear were followed by massive keloid formation. The association of arthrogryposis with the described ear and eye abnormalities and keloid formation appears to be due to a common pathogenetic mechanism.

Pulmonic stenosis was diagnosed since the report in 1972. The other infant in the original series of 4 cases also had an anomaly of vascular structures at the right base of the heart. This location of the congenital heart abnormalities is typical of Noonan syndrome and thus supports our original interpretation that the facial abnormalities seen in this case are indeed those of the XY-Turner phenotype, viz Noonan syndrome.

This syndrome is similar to one recently described by Pena et al and Punnett et al (J Pediatr 373-377, 1974) as "multiple ankyloses with facial anomalies and pulmonary hypoplasia." The spectrum of disorders appears to be wider than initially recognized because pulmonary hypoplasia is not obligatory (Pena and Shokeir, Birth Defects XII(5):201, 1976) and the disorder need not be lethal at birth. Inheritance appears to be autosomal recessive.

AN AUTOSOMAL DOMINANT FORM OF ARTHROGRYPOSIS MULTIPLEX CONGENITA (AMC) WITH UNUSUAL DERMATOGLYPHICS

Y. Lacassie, G. H. Sack, Jr., and V. A. McKusick

Division of Medical Genetics, Department of Medicine, The Johns Hopkins University School of Medicine, Baltimore, Maryland and Louisiana Heritable Disease Center, Department of Pediatrics, Louisiana State University Medical Center, New Orleans, Louisiana

AMC is characterized by congenital fixation of multiple joints. We report a father and daughter with similar clinical and dermatoglyphic findings suggesting autosomal dominant inheritance.

The father (39 years old) was born with absent flexion creases of fingers with limited flexion of all joints of upper limbs and neck. Talipes equinovarus was corrected by bilateral triple arthrodeses and later Achilles tendon extensions. He is now short with scoliosis and 4 symmetric dimples over posterior ilia. There is generalized limitation of gaze, especially upward, and atrophy of muscles of legs below knees. Intelligence is normal.

His 2-year-old daughter was born with flexion of hands, arms, and knees, dislocated hips, and bilateral talipes equinovarus. She is small, the neck is short with limited movement; no scoliosis; limited extension in all joints of upper limbs, hips, and knees; fixed equinovarus of ankles; bilateral dimples over sacrum; moderate generalized weakness of muscles, more prominent in lower limbs.

Both have normal nerve conduction velocities, muscle enzymes, histologic findings on muscle biopsy, and karyotypes. There are no other affected family members. The mother is normal.

Dermatoglyphic findings were abnormal and included: 1) in the fingers: a) high frequency of large size whorls with 3 triradii, b) high total ridge-count and pattern intensity, c) vertical orientation of ridges, d) accessory triradii over proximal phalanges, and e) absence of most flexion creases. 2) In the hands: a) lack of sharp delineation between fingers and palm with extra basal triradii, b) abnormal position of the axial triradii, c) simian crease, d) complete reverse main line orientation, most of the lines ending in the radial side of the palm (daughter only).

Information about dermatoglyphics in this syndrome is scarce because the flexion contractures of the fingers make the ridges difficult to interpret. The most frequent finding has been longitudinal alignment of the palmar ridges with main A lines ending in palmar areas 1 and 2. Bilateral, complete, or transitional simian creases and distal axial triradii with patterns on the hypothenar area also have been noted. Some of the clinical features in both patients may be explained as developmental anomalies due to the abnormal structure of the hands. However, others probably reflect an abnormal genotype. The unusual dermatoglyphics support the possibility that this represents a new syndrome of AMC.

PIEBALD TRAIT IN A RETARDED CHILD WITH INTERSTITIAL DELETION OF CHROMOSOME 4: A NEW SYNDROME

Y. Lacassie, T. F. Thurmon, and M. Tracy

Louisiana Heritable Disease Center, Department of Pediatrics, Louisiana State University School of Medicine in New Orleans, New Orleans, Louisiana

A 13-month-old girl with marked psychomotor retardation of development, pigmentary changes of the Piebald syndrome, abnormal dermatoglyphics, minor facial and hand malformations, and an interstitial deletion of the long arm of chromosome 4 [46,XX,del(4)(q11 q21)] is reported. The striking similarities with a case previously reported support the idea this is a new identifiable chromosomal syndrome. This syndrome could represent another case in which a mendelian trait is associated with a specific chromosomal deletion.

A NEW GROWTH DEFICIENCY SYNDROME WITH MUSCULAR HYPERTROPHY, JOINT LIMITATIONS, UNUSUAL FACIES AND MENTAL DEFICIENCY

S. A. Myhre, R. H. A. Ruvalcaba, and C. B. Graham

State of Washington, Department of Social and Health Services, Community Services Division, Rainier School, Buckley, Washington and Department of Pediatrics and Radiology, University of Washington, Seattle, Washington

Two strikingly similar unrelated male patients have the following pattern of anomalies: growth and mental deficiency, generalized muscular hypertrophy, joint limitations, unusual craniofacial appearance, hearing loss, and skeletal findings. The growth deficiency is of prenatal onset and has continued in the postnatal period with a normal rate of skeletal maturation. There is generalized muscular hypertrophy with decreased mobility in all joints. The craniofacial anomalies include hypoplasia of the maxilla, short philtrum, short palpebral fissures, and prognathism. Audiograms demonstrate a binaural, severe mixed hearing loss. The skeletal findings include a thickened calvarium, a prominent, broad mandible, shortened long and short tubular bones, hypoplastic iliac wings, broad ribs, and large, flattened nonbeaked vertebras with large pedicles. Older paternal age has been documented in these 2 cases.

THE WINDMILL VANE HAND SYNDROME IN A FATHER AND SON WITHOUT WHISTLING FACE

R. A. Norum, P. C. Klass, W. N. Lim, and M. W. Hilgartner

Departments of Medicine and Pediatrics, Cornell University Medical College, New York, New York

A 32-year-old man and his 8-month-old son had the same congenital bilateral hand deformities and clubbed feet. In both patients the hands showed contracture and ulnar deviation of the fingers at the metacarpophalangeal (MCP) joints. In the son the ulnar deviation was reducible, while in the father it was fixed. The thumbs were contracted at the MCP joints and adducted. Both patients had bilateral 4th finger palmar creases. Flexion of the wrists was absent in the son and limited to half the normal range in the father. Bilateral talipes equinovarus had been corrected surgically in both patients. There were no facial signs of the whistling face syndrome in either patient. The intercommissural distance was 54 mm in the father and 31 mm in the son. Growth has been normal in the son. The father's height was 170 cm. Neither patient has spine deformity, neck webbing, or hip contracture. Studies of clotting appeared to show a partial deficiency of factor 9 in both patients and abnormalities resembling von Willebrand disease in the son although neither has manifested a bleeding problem.

The son is the father's only child. The father's parents, sister, fraternal twin brother, a second brother, and that brother's 2 daughters and son all have no congenital hand or foot abnormalities. At the father's birth his father was 44 years old and his mother was 37.

The combination of hand and foot deformities without other signs of the whistling face syndrome suggests that these patients may have a distinct entity.

UNUSUAL ARTICULAR DYSPLASIAS WITH ASSOCIATED MALFORMATIONS

J. Perrin, E. Horrell, D. Corbett, J. Ryan, and H. Chen

Departments of Pediatrics, Radiology and Surgery, Wayne State University, Detroit, Michigan

Unusual failures of large joint formation (articular dysplasias) are presented in 3 unrelated patients with other uncommon conditions, including one with xeroderma pigmentosum.

Case 1, a patient with aplasia of knee joints and phocomelia of arms, was a 5-year-old female with 3 normal sibs. She presented as a foster child so pregnancy was unknown. She had a standing height of 79.45 cm (<3%) with a bilateral flexion ankylosis of the knees, absent patellas, popliteal pterygia, waddling gait, and hands attached to shoulders. Craniofacies and intelligence were normal. Roentgenograms, including technetium scan of the knees confirmed developmental fusion between well-formed distal femoral and proximal tibial epiphyses (complete absence of knee joints and patellas). In the upper limbs, forearm bones were absent, scapulas and humeri rudimentary, but there were 5 rays on each hand. The right kidney was ectopic.

Case 2 presented with aplasia of elbow joint and xeroderma pigmentosum. A 4-year-old male, he was the child of nonconsanguineous parents, the mother having vitiligo; 5 half sibs were normal. There was absent right ulna and total bony humeroradial ankylosis (absent elbow joint) and a hand with 2 radial metacarpals and 3 phalanges (bifid thumb). The left radius was shortened and dislocated at the elbow. The thumb was absent. He had xeroderma pigmentosum, photo-

phobia, narrow palpebral fissures and injected conjunctivas, generalized adeno-
pathy, and short stature.

   Case 3, a 9-year-old female with synarthrosis of elbow joints and club hands,
was born with bilateral 45° fixed elbows which lacked the olecranon process and
resembled knee joints on roentgenograms. Bilateral hand anomalies included radial
clubbing, soft tissue syndactyly, dorsal dislocations and flexion contractures of
MP and IP joints. She underwent numerous plastic procedures, as well as repeated
myringotomies for conductive hearing loss. Salient features at age 9 were normal
intelligence, esotropia, bilateral elbow synarthrosis, short fingers and short toes 2
and 3, and MP and IP flexion contractures. Her younger sister has scoliosis.

   Congenital absence or synarthrosis of large joints is rare, and we were unable
to find any report of the knee aplasia seen in *Case 1.* Joint malformations have
been associated with xeroderma pigmentosum (*Case 2*). *Case 3* had similar features to the autosomal dominant syndrome of bilateral elbow synostosis, brachydactyly, and carpal/tarsal fusions.

CONGENITAL PALATOPHARYNGEAL INCOMPETENCY: NOT ONE SYNDROME BUT TWO

S. Pruzansky, P. Parris, J. Laffer, S. Peterson-Falzone

Center for Craniofacial Anomalies, Abraham Lincoln School of Medicine, University of
Illinois at the Medical Center, Chicago, Illinois

   Congenital palatopharyngeal incompetency (CPI) is defined as incomplete
closure of the velopharyngeal port during speech in the absence of an overt cleft.
Although the entity has been recognized for more than 100 years, a comprehensive definition of the disorder, its etiology, mechanisms, and natural history remain to be elucidated. Review of more than 300 cases from a larger series in our
files confirmed the existence of at least 2 types of CPI. Type 1 had one or more
of a triad of visible stigmata such as bifid uvula, zone pellucida or diastasis of
the velar musculature, and submucous defect of the hard palate. Type 2 had no
such visible stigmata but demonstrated anomalies detectable on radiographic
examination which included short or thin velum, excessive pharyngeal depth,
anomalous cervical vertebras and craniovertebral junction, and platybasia. Family
studies indicate that the 2 types of CPI constitute separate genetic entities..

X-LINKED MENTAL DEFICIENCY ASSOCIATED WITH MEGALOTESTIS

R. H. A. Ruvalcaba, S. A. Myhre, E. C. Roosen-Runge, and J. B. Beckwith

State of Washington, Department of Social and Health Services, Community Services Division, Rainier School, Buckley, Washington and the Department of Pediatrics, Pathology and Biological Structure, University of Washington, Seattle, Washington

We have studied 2 families (Fa, Fb) that presented 7 males (4 of Fa, and 3 of Fb) with mental deficiency associated with megalotestis. The inheritance is suggestive of an X-linked recessive disorder. The severely affected males have been born to unaffected females, however, there are 2 females (1 of Fa, and 1 of Fb) who were mildly retarded and had severely affected sibs, and 1 female (Fa) who was mildly retarded and had no living male sibs. As the affected males produced no offspring, the possibility of male limited autosomal dominant inheritance cannot be ruled out. The birthweight for gestational age of the affected male subjects was above the 90th%. The endocrine studies were not conclusive.

Testicular biopsies showed edematous interstitium with tubules abnormally separated by a matrix in which collagen fibers were not abundant. Leydig cells appeared to be in minimal numbers. The seminiferous tubules contained spermatogenic cells at all stages of development. Morphometric and ultrastructural studies indicated an excess of interstitial and tubular fluid which was confirmed by analysis of dry vs wet weight.

A POSSIBLE NEW PREMATURE AGING SYNDROME

C. F. Salinas, R. J. Jorgenson, S. H. Schuman, S. D. Shapiro, and J. M. Goust

Department of Oral Medicine, Section of Clinical Genetics, Department of Family Practice, Department of Immunology and Microbiology, Medical University of South Carolina, Charleston, South Carolina

The purpose of this paper is to report an unusual case showing a constellation of congenital abnormalities that resembles the premature aging syndromes. However, the findings, to our knowledge, are not compatible with any of them. The proposita is a 14 8/12-year-old black male. He is the product of a 7-month pregnancy and his parents are reportedly not consanguineous. His mother at the time of his birth was 38 years old. She died in 1972 from "some sort of anemia," therefore, maternal and neonatal histories are uncertain. It was reported that another sib died early in life and was affected with characteristics similar to our patient.

Unusual physical features included the following findings: skeleton: microcephaly (45.8 cm), short stature, scoliosis, bilateral genu valgus, winging scapulas, asymmetric chest, bone fragility. Hair: greyish, sparse, fine with premature canities, absence of axillary and pubic hair. Skin: coarse, hyperkeratotic and parched with bleeding lesion at flexion creases. Severely involved are the hands, knees, elbows, and feet. Toes and fingertips are cool and devoid of pink color. Nails: fingernails and toenails ranged from hypoplastic to absent. Eyes: funduscopic examination reveals narrow, tortuous arterioles with silver wire appearance; no hemorrhages or exudates. Oral Cavity: smooth, depapillas and bluish pigmented tongue, absence of ruga palatina, discolored teeth, high incidence of caries (D.M.F. 16) and enlarged gingiva. Testes: cryptorchidism bilateral. Mental Development: retarded.

Other Clinical Findings: simian crease, low blood pressure (right arm 90/60 and left arm 80/40), reduced pulsation in dorsalis pedis and radial arteries bilaterally. Laboratory Findings: absence of sweat pores in the hand. Dental radiographs reveal a process of periodontosis with generalized periodontitis and abnormal morphology of the molars including taurodontia of the 2nd upper molars. Immunologic tests reveal that the absolute number of lymphocytes is normal. However, the total active rosette forming cells are markedly decreased (15.5% and 34% meanwhile, the normal values are 29% and 64%, respectively). Normal male karyotype, 46,XY.

DYSTONIA, NEURAL DEAFNESS AND POSSIBLE INTELLECTUAL IMPAIRMENT: A NEW FAMILIAL SYNDROME

N. Scribanu and C. Kennedy

Department of Pediatrics, Georgetown University Medical Center, Washington, DC

Dystonia has been reported as one of several neurologic symptoms in the syndrome referred to as atypical torsion dystonias (Eldrige, 1970). Deafness has been reported with several movement disorders (Herrmann et al, 1964; May et al, 1968; Latham et al, 1937). To our knowledge, dystonia with neural deafness has not been previously reported. The familial pattern suggesting X-linked inheritance has not been seen before the report of dystonia in males from the Island of Panay, Philippines (Lee et al, 1975). Recently we have studied a family exhibiting all these features. The proband was seen by us for the first time at the age of 8 years at which time he presented with: a) deafness; b) severe dysarthria; c) striking deterioration of the handwriting; d) occasional bizarre posture of his head and neck; and e) hyperactive behavior. The pregnancy, perinatal period, and early growth and development were described as normal. A sensorineural hearing loss was confirmed by audiometric testing at the age of 2 years at which time the patient was fitted with a hearing aid and given speech therapy which later enabled him to start school in a special class. At 7 years of age he started to present increasing distortions of his handwriting and dystonic movements of his left hand and neck; by the age of 9 years he was confined to a wheelchair with severe retrocollis and was unable to articulate at all. He had a brief period of clinical improvement under a trial therapy with L-DOPA after which he continued to deteriorate and died at the age of 11 years. The patient's parents are clinically normal, but the mother's youngest brother is said to have had an onset of deafness at the age of 6 years after which he developed progressive dystonic posturing and died in his 20s. The patient's brother is 19 years old and in good health. A sister is 26 years old and well. Her 6-year-old son was born prematurely at 7 months. He thrived poorly, has severe bilateral sensorineural hearing loss, failure of normal language development, and severe psychomotor retardation. The pathologic examination of the brain revealed neuronal loss and gliosis in both caudate nuclei putamen and globus pallidus. The temporal bone histopathology revealed severe degeneration of the sensory epithelium and supporting cells in the basal turn of the cochlea. The organ of Corti was absent.

In summary, we have described a progressive, familial movement disorder, the characteristic features of which are dystonia preceded by progressive sensorineural hearing loss. Intellectual impairment may also be an intrinsic part of the syndrome. The X-linked recessive mode of inheritance has been considered on the basis that 3 males were affected in 3 consecutive generations (if one considers the presence of deafness in the 6-year-old boy who represents the 3rd generation). The patient's mother, maternal grandmother, and patient's sister are clinically unaffected.

THE TWO FACES OF TRISOMY 13

L. R. Shapiro, P. L. Wilmot, A. S. Lustenberger, and P. A. Duncan

Letchworth Village Developmental Center, Thiells, New York and Departments of Pediatrics and Pathology, Westchester County Medical Center and New York Medical College, Valhalla, New York

In 1966, Snodgrass classified the D trisomy syndrome into 2 phenotypic categories according to facial appearance. Category 1 patients have holoprosencephaly associated with cleft lip and palate, orbital hypotelorism, severe ocular abnormalities, hypoplasia of the crista galli, and portions of the ethmoid bone and nasal septum. Category 2 patients do not resemble Category 1 patients, but do resemble each other. There is no cleft lip and/or palate and the nose is bulbous. There are no severe optic or orbital defects.

Prior to the advent of chromosomal banding techniques, autoradiographic studies suggested that different D-group chromosome trisomies might account for the phenotypic variation. With the advent of chromosomal banding techniques, specific identification of the trisomic D-group chromosomes is now possible. A patient with the Snodgrass Category 2 facies and clinical diagnosis of trisomy D was found to have trisomy 13 confirmed by the Giemsa banding technique.

Review of the literature revealed that this is only the third case of Snodgrass Category 2 facies confirmed by banding techniques to be trisomy 13, and one of the previous cases had been confused with the Rubinstein-Taybi syndrome. The explanation of phenotypic variation within trisomy 13 is not clear and is further confounded by the fact that Category 1 facies may occur as an isolated finding with no chromosomal aberration.

A SYNDROME OF SHORT STATURE AND RECURRENT LOWER LIMB ULCERATION PROBABLY INHERITED AS AN X-LINKED RECESSIVE TRAIT

I. Shine, R. Levine, and G. Carlson

Thomas Hunt Morgan Institute of Genetics, Lexington, Kentucky

Four male members of one family from early childhood to their mid-thirties had recurrent stasis type ulceration of the lower legs which rarely healed despite all forms of conventional therapy including repeated skin grafts, 2 years continuous hospitalization, and amputation for one member. The familial distribution of the affected members is consistent with X-linked recessive inheritance.

THE STIFF SKIN SYNDROME: NEW GENETIC AND BIOCHEMICAL INVESTIGATIONS

H. Singer, D. Valle, J. Rogers, and G. Thomas

Departments of Neurology and Pediatrics, Johns Hopkins Hospital, Baltimore, Maryland

The stiff skin syndrome (SS) is a presumed autosomal dominantly inherited disorder characterized by thick, hard skin, limitation of joint mobility, and firm muscles. These clinical features plus histochemical studies of the affected skin and cultured fibroblasts of 3 previously reported cases have suggested an abnormality of glycosaminoglycan (GAG) metabolism in SS (Esterly and McKusick, 1969).

We now report a new family with affected members in 4 successive generations plus an affected offspring of a previously reported case. Histochemical and biochemical studies on these patients failed to confirm an abnormality of GAG metabolism.

Cases 1 and *2: Case 1* is a 7-year-old white female whose skin appears normal but is hard, thick, and immobile. Nodular cutaneous thickenings are present over the metacarpophalangeal joints and there is limitation of extension of the fingers and elbows. The muscles although very firm have normal strength. Slit-lamp exam is normal and the patient's IQ is 110. Her father, *Case 2,* is a 39-year-old accountant whose nonprogressive physical findings are similar to his daughter's. His sisters, father, and grandfather are reported to have similar physical findings.

Case 3: Case 3 is a 3-month-old white male whose father, *Case 4,* has been previously reported as a case of SS. This infant has a normal exam except for thick hard skin most pronounced over the shoulders and upper limbs.

Laboratory Investigation: Histochemical examination of skin biopsies from *Case 1* and *Case 2* was normal as was a muscle biopsy from *Case 1.* Activity of the lysosomal enzyme arylsulfatase A was normal in the serum of *Case 2* and *Case 1* excluding mucolipidosis III. Cultured fibroblasts S^{35} incorporation kinetics were measured on *Case 2, Case 1,* and *Case 4.* Total S^{35} incorporation and chase with unlabeled media was normal. Activity of several lysosomal enzymes was within normal limits. Reduced levels (40% of normal) of α-fucosidase were demonstrated in *Case 1* and *Case 2* fibroblasts, however, the α-fucosidase activity of *Case 4* was clearly in the normal range.

Demonstration of affected members in successive generations in 2 families proves that the SS syndrome is inherited as an autosomal dominant. No evidence for a specific lysomal enzyme defect has been found. We speculate that a defect of collagen or proteoglycans may be the biochemical abnormality in this syndrome.

FAMILIAL MULTIPLE GLOMUS TUMORS

C. Sirinavin and E. W. Lovrien

The Crippled Children's Division and Medical Genetics, University of Oregon Health Sciences Center, Portland, Oregon

Multiple glomus tumors are benign skin tumors rarely described in contrast to the well-recognized painful solitary glomus tumor. Evaluation of a child with multiple glomus tumors (MGT) subsequently led to identification of 28 affected individuals in a 5-generation kindred in which 126 members were examined. Twenty-five living individuals had 287 MGT with 64 tumors in one individual. Of those affected, 17 were male and 11 female with an age range of 3–79 years.

In 4 individuals MGT had been present since birth and in 12 cases they appeared after birth but before age 15. Fifty-eight percent were located on the upper limbs, 21% lower limbs, 10.5% trunk, and 10.5% head and neck. Of the 97 MGT on the hands, only 9 were on the distal phalanges. The appearance of the tumors was round, domed, well-circumscribed with 85% blue, 10% purple, and 5% red. The largest MGT was 20 x 20 x 6 mm; only 10% were greater than 10 mm. The appearance of the tumors was consistent with an autosomal dominant pattern of inheritance. One girl had MGT without an affected parent suggesting incomplete penetrance. There were no consistent associated illnesses. Electron microscopy showed the glomus cells to resemble smooth muscle cells. The tumor was noncapsulated with numerous dilated endothelial-lined vascular channels surrounded by glomus cells. MGT can be microscopically distinguished from solitary glomus tumors which are not usually familial, and which usually occur in females. The nature of MGT suggests a hamartoma. The familial manifestation may be the result of the 2-mutation theory (proposed by Knudson) with a germinal mutation inherited from a parent followed by a somatic mutation in affected members.

X-LINKED DUCHENE MUSCULAR DYSTROPHY IN A FEMALE WITH XO/XX MOSAICISM

M. H. K. Shokeir, E. J. Ives, and K. L. Ying

Section of Medical Genetics, University of Saskatchewan University Hospital, Saskatoon, Canada

A sibship with 2 children (a brother and sister) who are affected with Duchene muscular dystrophy is presented. Chromosome studies conducted on lymphocytes and skin fibroblasts from 2 locations, thigh and abdomen, revealed X-chromosome mosaicism with 42%, 53%, and 56% of the cells with sex chromosomal complement of XO, whereas 58%, 47%, and 44% of the nuclei had normal XX complement respectively. The diagnosis of muscular dystrophy was confirmed clinically, biochemically, histologically, and by electromyography. The severity of affliction in the sister (who is 2 years younger) is comparable to that of her affected older brother at the corresponding age. Serum enzyme studies suggested that both the mother and maternal grandmother are heterozygous carriers.

Severity of further involvement and ultimate prognosis in the sister will likely depend on the proportion of the XO cell line and that of the paternal X-inactivated nuclei in her muscle cells. Although the former may be surmised from the data on mosaicism obtained from other tissues, the latter remains obscure.

ANIRIDIA, MENTAL RETARDATION AND GENITAL ABNORMALITY IN TWO PATIENTS WITH 46,XY,11p−

A. C. M. Smith, E. Sujansky, and V. M. Riccardi

Department of Biophysics and Genetics, University of Colorado Medical Center, Denver, Colorado, Department of Pediatrics, Milwaukee Children's Hospital, Milwaukee, Wisconsin

We describe 2 cases with a partial deletion of the short arms of chromosome No. 11, which suggests a new chromosome syndrome. Both patients had mental retardation, aniridia, and abnormal external genitalia, consisting of 2nd degree hypospadias in one patient and ambiguous genitalia in the other. Chromosome analysis performed on one of these individuals prior to the availability of differential staining techniques was interpreted as normal.

The excessive occurrence of Wilms tumor in patients with certain congenital defects has been reported. The association of Wilms tumor with aniridia, mental and growth retardation, microcephaly, genitourinary anomalies, and deformities of pinna represents a well-defined syndrome the etiology of which is not understood. Common teratogenic and oncogenic mechanisms have been postulated. Normal chromosome analysis using conventional staining techniques was reported in 5 cases. The utilization of differential staining techniques might detect a chromosome abnormality in some of the previously described cases. Since children with the autosomal dominant form of aniridia do not show an increased incidence of Wilms tumor, individuals with 11p− may represent a subgroup of aniridia patients who have an increased potential for the development of Wilms tumor.

Our finding of ambiguous genitalia in patients with a deletion involving the short arm of chromosome No. 11 emphasizes that pseudohermaphroditism can on occasion result from aberrations of autosomes. Therefore, the buccal smear is not always sufficient in the evaluation of patients with ambiguous genitalia.

THE MAJEWSKI SYNDROME − A CASE REPORT

A. Sommer, A. Mulne, and L. Cordero

Department of Pediatrics, College of Medicine, Ohio State University, Children's Hospital, Columbus, Ohio

Majewski has described a form of lethal neonatal dwarfism with specific combination of short ribs and limbs, polydactyly, syndactyly, median cleft lip, genital anomalies, and anomalies of visceral organs. To date, there are few reports in English literature of this condition.

The present case, *Case 1,* was a newborn black female born to a 12-year-old mother with no previous medical problems. Consanguinity between the parents was denied. The patient was delivered by C-section and was immediately noted to have respiratory distress, which appeared due in part to a small thoracic cage. Further examination revealed a relatively large head with frontal prominence, depressed nasal bridge, low-set ears, cleft lip, cleft palate, cleft tongue, and hypoglossia. Extreme shortening of all limbs was predominant with polydactyly and syndactyly present. Death occurred within 24 hours due to decreased thoracic expansion and respiratory distress. At autopsy further findings included short ribs with hypoplasia of the lungs, ASD with right ventricular enlargement, agenesis of the gallbladder and left adrenal, mobile cecum with shortening of the small bowel, accessory spleen, and cerebral edema and congestion. Histologic examination showed excess cartilage with little osteoid in very coarse trabecular, irregular epiphyseal plates with distorted chondroblasts, diminished bone marrow spaces with extramedullary hematopoiesis present in the liver, and cystic changes in the kidney. Although Majewski syndrome had many features in common with other forms of short ribbed dwarfism, including ATD, CED, Saldino-Noonan syndrome, and Meckel syndrome, the severe shortening of all limbs, early mortality, and cleft lip and palate appear to place this patient in the category of the Majewski syndrome.

THE OTO-PALATO-DIGITAL SYNDROME

R. S. Stanwick and R. I. Macpherson

Departments of Pediatrics and Radiology, University of Manitoba, Winnipeg, Manitoba, Canada

The oto-palato-digital syndrome (Dudding et al, 1967) is a skeletal dysplasia consisting of short stature, characteristic facies, and unusual deformities of the hands and feet. Cleft palate, conductive deafness, and other congenital malformations are inconsistent features of the disorder. A pattern of radiologic features involving the skull, spine, hands, and feet is diagnostic of the syndrome. Twenty-six affected females and 23 affected males in 5 consecutive generations of one kindred and 2 affected females and 2 affected males in 3 generations of a second kindred were studied. The clinical and radiologic features tend to be most striking in affected males. Affected females exhibit the same features, but usually less pronounced. None of the 13 male offspring of affected males exhibited any stigmata of the syndrome. These findings suggest that the mode of inheritance is most likely X-linked dominant with an intermediate expression in the female.

AN ASSOCIATION OF AORTICOTRUNCOCONAL ABNORMALITIES, VELOPALATINE INCOMPETENCE, AND UNUSUAL CERVICAL SPINE FUSION

A. M. Stern, J. M. Sigmann, B. L. Perry, L. R. Kuhns and A. K. Poznanski

Departments of Pediatrics and Radiology, University of Michigan Medical Center, Ann Arbor, Michigan

Twenty-six patients were seen in cardiology with congenital heart defects and velopalatine incompetence (VPI). The cardiovascular defects were primarily of aorticotruncoconal origin (tetralogy of Fallot 14, ventricular septal defect 9, truncus arteriosus 3) though additional anomalies were seen. Fluoroscopically the VPI appeared to result from shortening and poor motion of the soft palate. All patients had high-arched palates. Only 2 children had small clefts of the soft palate and none had a cleft lip. Most of the patients had characteristic facies consisting of down-turned mouths, malocclusion, flattening of the zygomatic region, and dystopia canthorum. Twenty-two had small, deformed pinnas. Eleven had head circumferences which were 2 or more standard deviations below normal, and 13 were mildly mentally retarded. Two children had severe hypothyroidism and also tetany of the newborn period. Unusual posterior fusion of C_2 and C_3 was found in 10 of 20 patients having cervical spine radiographs. As a rule of the anterior arch of C_1 was large and the posterior arch unusually small. Umbilical hernias occurred in 14 patients and inguinal hernias in 5. Ten had tapering fingers.

Many of these characteristics have been seen in the DiGeorge syndrome and other branchial developmental disturbances. The patients described herein appear to be related to the above syndromes though none of those studied presented with definite immune deficiencies. The syndrome appears to be sporadic since no affected family members were found and there was no history of consanguinity in the parents.

PARTIAL 18-TRISOMY DUE TO 9-18 TRANSLOCATION

R. L. Summitt, R. S. Wilroy, Jr., P. A. Martens, and P. A. Wilkerson

University of Tennessee Center for the Health Sciences, Memphis, Tennessee

A white female infant, birthweight 2,637 gm, had hypotonia, abnormal ears, capillary hemangioma of the forehead, narrow palate, micrognathia, ptergyium colli, prominent heels, overlapping fingers without camptodactyly, and no digital arch patterns. Chromosomal analysis prior to availability of banding techniques revealed a metacentric chromosome replacing a chromosome of the C group.

This was interpreted initially as a presumptive isochromosome of the long arm of X. Although the infant thrived, mental and developmental retardation became evident.

When the patient was 8 years old a chromosomal analysis, using banding techniques, revealed a karyotype of 46,XX,der(9),rcp(9:18)p24;q12) with trisomy for the distal long arm of chromosome 18, a product of adjacent-1 segregation of a maternally derived balanced reciprocal translocation. The same balanced translocation 46,XX,rcp(9:18)(q24:q12), was detected in the proband's brother, maternal aunt, first cousins, grandmother, and great-grandmother.

Four women who carry the balanced translocation have conceived 14 times. Four of these pregnancies have produced normal individuals with normal karyotypes. Six offspring are the products of alternate segregation of the translocation and thus also carry the balanced translocation while only one person, the proband, is the product of adjacent segregation. Interestingly, 3 pregnancies terminated in spontaneous abortions. This case suggests that patients who are partially trisomic for the distal long arm of chromosome 18 may have less severe mental retardation and milder phenotypic abnormalities than those who have complete 18-trisomy.

SEGREGATION OF AN INSERTIONAL CHROMOSOMAL REARRANGEMENT IN THREE GENERATIONS

K. Toomey, T. Mohandas, R. Sparkes, M. Kaback, and D. Rimoin

Divisions of Medical Genetics, Harbor General Hospital Campus and Center for Health Sciences, UCLA School of Medicine, Los Angeles, California

Translocations involving direct insertions between 2 chromosomes are estimated to occur in one in 5,000 births. We wish to report such a rearrangement segregating in 3 generations. The proband, a female referred for microcephaly, mental retardation, short stature, and expressive aphasia also exhibited hypertelorism, a wide down-turning mouth, short neck with a broad back, bilateral single flexion creases of the 5th digits, and abnormal stance with flexion at the hips and knees. A maternal uncle and great uncle possess similar dysmorphic features and speech difficulties. Cytogenetic analysis of the proband using Q-banding technique revealed a deletion of band 13q21→13q22. In the mother, maternal grandmother and 2 male sibs, the deleted segment was inserted into the proximal portion of the long arm of chromosome 3. The balanced carrier is thus, 46,XX or XY,inv ins(3;13)(q12;q22q21) ("Paris Conference (1971),"

Birth Defects: Orig Art Ser, 8(7):1–43, 1971.) The proband is deficient for
13(q21→q22) and presents a phenotype similar to previous reports of interstitial
q13 deletions enabling further delineation of the 13q- syndromes. Gene marker
studies are in progress.

A SYNDROME ASSOCIATED WITH INTERSTITIAL DELETION
OF CHROMOSOME 7q

H. Valentine and F. Sergovich

Department of Paediatrics, University of Western Ontario and Children's Psychiatric
Research Institute, London, Ontario, Canada

The first and only child of a 29-year-old mother and 28-year-old father, born
6 weeks prematurely with a birthweight of 2,100 gm, was recognized at birth as
abnormal. He was extremely thin with profuse scalp hair, anteverted nostrils,
low-set ears, a partial facial palsy, undescended testes, rocker-bottom feet and
clinical pulmonary stenosis.

At 7 months of age there was microcephaly, a long upper lip, hypotonia,
dorsiflexion of both great toes, a transverse palmar crease on one hand and 10
digital whorl patterns. Psychomotor development was at the 2 month level
(photographs in the first week and at intervals thereafter are on record).

Myoclonic jerks of all limbs have been observed. The electroencephalogram
shows multiple independent spikes maximal in both parietal and occipital regions.

Peripheral blood leukocyte culture showed no abnormality on "solid" staining but fluorescent analysis indicated deletion of a small portion of chromosome
No. 7. The interpretation of the analysis is of deletion of the band area q11, q22,
ie 46,XY del (7) (q11q12). The chromosome analyses of both parents are normal.

Quinacrine fluorescent staining of 290 consecutive blood cultures in a routine
hospital laboratory revealed 3 variants: an elongated constriction on No. 9 (which
had been noted on regular staining), a pericentric inversion of the constriction
on No. 9 in the young mother of a child with Down syndrome, and inversion of
the centromere region of No. 3 in a French Canadian child with frontonasal dysplasia.

In a population of 100 moderately to profoundly retarded persons, 2 examples
of an inversion in No. 3 were found in 2 unrelated children of French Canadian
parentage. It may be that the inversion in No. 3 is a not uncommon variant among
persons of French Canadian descent.

The revelation by fluorescents of a significant chromosome abnormality un-
detected by conventional staining has been, for this laboratory, a unique event.
It would not have come to light had not the parents, persistent in their demands

for an explanation of the defect in their child, put pressure on the clinician, who passed the pressure along to the cytogeneticist.

PARTIAL TETRASOMY 15 SYNDROME DUE TO A BISATELLITED ISOCHROMOSOME

D. L. Van Dyke, M. Logan, L. Weiss, and G. S. Pai

Henry Ford Hospital, Detroit, Michigan

A 5-year-old boy of Arabian descent was karyotyped because he had moderate mental retardation, severe speech retardation, hyperactivity, strabismus, and an abnormal EEG.

Three cell lines were identified in preparations of 104 cells obtained from peripheral blood cultures. A normal karyotype was observed in 30 cells; 54 cells had an extra E-group-sized submetacentric chromosome with satellites on both the long and short arms. The remaining 20 cells each had, in addition to the first marker (M1), a second bisatellited chromosome (M2) which was the smallest chromosome in the karyotype. This smaller marker was morphologically similar to the small extra bisatellited chromosomes seen occasionally in phenotypically normal individuals. Since both ends of M1 and M2 were satellited and participated in acrocentric associations, the markers were derived from one or more acrocentric chromosomes.

C-banding demonstrated that both markers were dicentric. However, M1 had only one primary constriction. Therefore one centromere was apparently inactive, analogous to that seen in certain tandem X-X translocations and X isochromosomes. Although low frequency mosaicism cannot be excluded, the parents did not appear to carry either marker. Genotyping and karyotyping data were consistent with paternity.

We therefore suggest that the dicentric M1 was derived from meiotic breakage and sister chromatid fusion in the proximal long arm of an acrocentric chromosome. This would have produced a symmetric isodicentric chromosome, plus 1 or 2 acentric fragments. M2 then could have resulted from a dicentric bridge-break-synthesis-reunion phenomenon. G-, C-, and Q-banding data are consistent with the isodicentric having originated from a chromosome 15.

Similar phenotypic and karyotypic findings have been described in 3 other patients (Crandall et al, Am J Ment Defic 77:571-78, 1973; and Parker and Alfi, Lancet 1, 1972-1973). In 2 patients a bisatellited chromosome indistinguishable from our M1 was observed in all of 30 metaphases, but was interpreted as having originated from a translocation between a chromosome 15 and another acrocentric. In one patient the extra chromosome was said to represent a trisomy for the proximal half of chromosome 15. All 4 subjects had normal height, weight, and head circumference. Abnormalities present were hyperactivity (4/4), mental retardation (4/4), abnormalities of speech (3/3), strabismus (3/4), EEG abnormalities (3/3), increased number of ulnar loops (2/3), and hypotonia (2/3). The frequency of this partial tetrasomy 15 syndrome may be greater than presently recognized because individuals with mental retardation in association with a superfically normal phenotype are frequently not karyotyped.

DUPLICATION 10q SYNDROME (q22→qter)

J. J. Yunis and R. C. Lewandowski, Jr.

Medical Genetics Division, Department of Laboratory Medicine and Pathology, University of Minnesota Medical School, Minneapolis, Minnesota

In 1974, Yunis and Sanchez described 4 cases with partial trisomy 10q. Since then, 13 additional cases have been studied, making possible the detailed characterization of this new chromosome disorder. These patients represent a distinct clinical syndrome with unique facial features and unusual somatic anomalies, particularly of the hands and feet. The constellation of facial features is pathognomonic and include a spacious forehead, oval and flat-appearing face, arched and wide-spread eyebrows, slight antimongoloid slants, small palpebral fissures, microphthalmia, small nose with anteverted nostrils and flat nasal bridge, prominent malar areas, bow-shaped mouth with prominent upper lip, micrognathia, malformed and/or low-set ears. Most patients had defects of hands and feet. The most commonly found anomalies include camptodactyly, proximally implanted thumbs and/or great toes, a wide space between 1st and 2nd toes, and bilateral syndactyly between 2nd and 3rd toes. Approximately one-third of all patients showed deep plantar furrows. Common trunk anomalies include short neck, heart defects, and cryptorchidism (7/12 males). The patients commonly demonstrate microcephaly, marked psychomotor retardation, and severe hypotrophy. In this syndrome, there appears to be a preponderance of affected males (12/17) and all but one case resulted from a familial balanced translocation. Most of the patients are trisomic for the distal half (q23→qter) or distal third (q24→qter) of the long arm of chromosome 10. The prognosis is poor since about half of the patients die before the first year of life and those surviving are bedridden cripples unable to communicate.

PHENOTYPE-KARYOTYPE CORRELATIONS IN 76 PATIENTS WITH THE TURNER SYNDROME

R. S. Wilroy, R. L. Summitt, P. R. Martens, T. T. Avirachan, and R. E. Tipton

Departments of Pediatrics, Anatomy, and the Child Development Center, University of Tennessee Center for the Health Sciences, Memphis, Tennessee

This report describes the phenotypes and karyotypes of 76 patients with the Turner syndrome evaluated by the Genetics Unit of the University of Tennessee Center for the Health Sciences. Their karyotypes are as follows:

43 patients: 45,X
8 patients: 45,X/46,XX
1 patient : 45,X/47,XXX
4 patients: 46,X,i(Xq)
1 patient : 46,X,i(Xq)/46,X,del(X)(q11)
5 patients: 45,X/46,X,i(Xq)
4 patients: 46,XXq-
1 patient : 45,X/46,X,r(X)
7 patients: 45,X/46,X,mar
2 patients: 45,X/46,XY

Of the 43 individuals with apparent complete sex chromosome monosomy, a single patient developed a gonadoblastoma in one dysgenetic gonad and a fibrocystadenoma in the other. Polycystic ovarian disease was detected in one patient with karyotype 45,X/46,XX.

Gonadoblastomas were found in 2 other patients, one with karyotype 45,X/46,X?del(Y) and one with karyotype 45,X/46,XY. In the latter, only 46 XY cells were found in lymphocytes and skin fibroblasts; only in fibroblasts cultured from the streak gonad was 45,X/46,XY mosaicism found.

Our findings suggest that chromosomal analyses be performed on multiple tissues in all patients with the Turner syndrome, especially in those with signs of virilization or who feminize at puberty. This is not only for the purpose of diagnostic confirmation, but also in an effort to detect a minor Y-bearing cell line. Further, our findings suggest that exploratory laparotomy with gonadal biopsy be performed on any patient with the Turner syndrome who exhibits masculinization or who feminizes at puberty, regardless of the karyotype.

Index